## NOTE TO USERS

This information is considered by B.C. Cancer Agency staff to offer clear, general information concerning cancer care which will help to answer frequently asked questions. However, in some instances, it may contain treatment or related information which varies from Agency practice.

This material is not intended to replace advice given by your physician or other health care providers. If you have any questions or would like more current information or further guidance, you are encouraged to speak to your cancer specialist, other Clinic staff or your personal physician.

# Comprehensive
# Cancer Care

# Comprehensive Cancer Care

## Integrating Alternative, Complementary, and Conventional Therapies

*James S. Gordon, M.D.*
*Sharon Curtin*

PERSEUS PUBLISHING
*Cambridge, Massachusetts*

Library of Congress Catalog Card Number: 00-102288

ISBN: 0–7382–0284-3
Copyright © 2000 by James S. Gordon, M.D., and Sharon Curtin

Perseus Publishing is a member of the Perseus Books Group.

Text design by Cynthia Young
Set in 11-point Sabon by the Perseus Books Group

1 2 3 4 5 6 7 8 9 10—03 02 01 00
First printing, May 2000

Perseus Publishing books are available at special discounts for bulk purchases in the United States by corporations, institutions, and other organizations. For more information, please contact the Special Markets Department at HarperCollins Publishers, 10 East 53rd Street, New York, NY 10022, or call 1–212–207–7528.

Find us on the World Wide Web at http://www.perseusbooks.com

*To those living and dying with cancer who have taught us so much about courage, candor, generosity, suffering, and the richness of being human.*

# Contents

# Acknowledgments

OUR EDUCATION IN cancer care has been intensive and ongoing. The people whose stories we tell in this book—the men, women, and children with cancer—have been the primary reason for it. There have been many guides along the way. Some of the most important are Henry Dreher, William Fair, M.D., Mike Hawkins, M.D., Michael Lerner, Ph.D., Ralph Moss, Ph.D., and Mary Ann Richardson, D.P.H.

The Comprehensive Cancer Care conferences began with a conversation with Center for Mind-Body Medicine board member Fera Simone and her husband Arman. They and others have made contributions that have made it possible for the Center to put on these conferences. Jane Blaustein in particular helped us to put transcripts of the conferences on our Web site and begin the groundwork for this book.

The National Cancer Institute and the National Institutes of Health have been particularly helpful in supporting these conferences. Wayne Jones, M.D., the Director of the Office of Alternative Medicine, gave initial encouragement, and William Harlan, M.D., the Acting Director of the new National Center for Complementary and Alternative Medicine, continued it. Richard Klausner, M.D., the Director of the National Cancer Institute, Robert Wittes, M.D., Deputy Director, and Jeffrey White, M.D., the Director of NCI's Office of Cancer Complementary and Alternative Medicine, have consistently supported our efforts. When he became director of NCCAM, Steven Straus, M.D., saw the importance of the meeting and enlarged the NCCAM participation.

All of these people have generously participated in and helped us to shape these conferences. So, too, has David Rosenthal, M.D., a past president of the American Cancer Society and the chair of the ACS Committee on Complementary and Alternative Therapies.

The small staff of the Center for Mind-Body Medicine has been responsible for the large, even Herculean, effort necessary to put on these conferences. We're grateful to all of them, and particularly to Carol Goldberg, M.A. LCSW, who helped us organize the first two conferences, and to Marty Cathcart and Susan Lord, M.D., who helped plan the agendas and bring the participants together.

Chris Tomasino, our agent, and Marnie Cochran, our editor at Perseus, moved heaven and earth—and us as well—to get the book out before Comprehensive Cancer Care 2000. We would hardly have been able to finish this book—and certainly not have been able to do it in a timely fashion—without the support of Klia Bassing, Tina Linden, and Catalina Talero.

Last, but certainly not least, we are indebted to Hala Azzam, Kate Bosch, Sabrina Malkani, and Glennie Rabin, who did research, worked on the manuscript, and provided useful criticism, good humor, and relentless encouragement.

# Introduction

IN THE NEXT few years, cancer will surpass heart disease as the number one cause of death in the United States. Every year, more than 1.2 million Americans will be diagnosed with cancer, joining the 8 million who are presently living with the disease. Statistically, cancer is as common as acne and as ubiquitous as male-pattern baldness.

Cancer is characterized by a process of uncontrollable growth. One cell receives a molecular message that begins a perversion of the most basic function of life, cell growth and division. If this "renegade cell" evades the body's normal surveillance and control mechanisms it begins a process of malignant transformation. Instead of contributing to vital cooperative functioning of the organism, cancer is the wild development of cellular structures with only one aim: to multiply and expand.

In our bodies, this process goes on for many months, years, or even decades before the uncontrolled cell division has developed the size and power to cause symptoms. In this way, cancer is a gradually unfolding biological event. But the diagnosis of cancer by an oncologist, or cancer specialist, is usually sudden and unexpected. For the cancer patient it is a personal and immediate marker of transformation, the beginning of a painful and profound process of change.

## Martin's Story

One night, almost 20 years ago, Martin had a grand mal seizure, crashing to the floor like a fallen monument. He was hit by an inner electrical storm, a chaotic circuitry flashing through his brain. One minute, he was plotting journalistic coups and exposing wickedness;

the next, he woke up with his wife crying, his head shaved and drilled, the doctors silent but shaking their heads, and the room smelling of fear.

Martin was barely 50, a big, greedy, loud, Irish storyteller. He was our friend, and he had brain cancer.

Martin created chaos and surprises wherever he went. He never seemed to hesitate, retreat, or avoid an interesting experience. He used his mind as a weapon, his tongue like a laser, throwing puns, insights, brilliant ideas, and bad jokes in all directions. His eyes were that deceptive, soft, Irish blue, animated by intelligence and malice. When he moved, you realized how big his bones were, and he defined every space he occupied. Charismatic, brilliant, and mocking, from the beginning he saw the irony in this aggressive malignant growth in his brain and the devastating consequences of treatment.

His hair, once straw colored and thick, grew back a soft, gentle white. By that time he was ready to go home. Hospitals are boring once you've intimidated the staff and broken most of the rules. The food is awful, sex is forbidden, and it's hard to have a good conversation in that antiseptic atmosphere. Martin also knew his tumor was not responding to treatment.

Jane, his wife, understood. She made arrangements, converting a downstairs sunroom into a sickroom. *My daughter's lending me her playroom*, Martin said. *I'll be haunted by the ghosts of all those mutilated Barbie dolls and ambushed by dinosaurs. But I'll be home, and we can have martinis before dinner and I can write without some fool requiring my cooperation.*

Martin was a realist, and also a poet. He had a very strong sense of who he was and how he controlled his own narrative. He wanted to continue to write and to live his own story. So he came home, and Jane began long hours of coordinating his care. All that was needed was the cooperation of the entire health care machine, including ambulance drivers, five doctors, the insurance company, the equipment rental company, pharmacies, the nurses, and a rotating group of home care workers, not to mention their daughter's school, Jane's boss, and the friends and relatives who wanted to help.

Chaos ruled, of course, and Murphy's law held: Whatever could go wrong, did. *Improvise*, Martin would roar, *that's what life, good medicine, and music are all about, creative improvisation!* He didn't care about the details or the hardship on others; he insisted on being Martin.

The burden of care fell on Jane. She was the juggler, catching the balls thrown by Martin, his illness, the doctors, hired caregivers who sometimes neglected to show up, and relatives who appeared without warning. Somehow, she managed to keep everything moving and finesse the misfires. The strain and stress showed. Martin would blame her for the least perceived neglect, friends gave thoughtless advice unaccompanied by offers of help, their daughter became more demanding. The paraphernalia required for home care began to take over the house. Jane and their daughter felt they had one little corner, one safe place, in an upstairs bedroom. There they could hide, brushing each other's hair, talking about school, and as time went on, they would sleep curled together like puppies.

We sat for hours listening to Martin. At first we thought he wanted our help in exploring complementary therapies. We were ready with books and meditation tapes and menu plans; we brought over bottles of herbs and supplements. We suggested people who could help with massage and guided imagery. Martin listened and nodded and agreed with us about immune enhancement and let us treat him once or twice with acupuncture, but he had another agenda.

Martin wanted us to listen. He already knew that trying to assign blame for his cancer was a useless enterprise. He faced his cancer, and his death, with his eyes open, denying nothing. He required the same courage and forthrightness from us. Simplistic answers wouldn't do. Palliative care was useful—he accepted massage as well as the morphine that eased his pain—but he was looking for something else, and the force of his desire was awesome to behold.

This was a man of thought and words, and he wanted—needed—a way to think about his cancer. He saw this as the final piece in his story, and he approached this search as he did everything, dedicated to the truth of the experience, groping for the important words, trying and discarding ideas.

Martin talked about the history of disease and medicine. He knew the great stories of simple solutions ignored—such as washing hands between patients to prevent the spread of infection—and the complicated treatments that failed, from bloodletting to modern surgical procedures. He talked about the power of serendipity in scientific discovery and the force of the shaman's curse. He knew about placebo response and faith healers and how the mind could alter every function in the physical body. We laughed and we argued. Martin was an opinionated, self-absorbed man. Spending one or eight hours with him was exhausting and frustrating and stimulating. He was searching for a place to stand and face his cancer. When we finally understood his purpose, we saw that he was writing his story, his own journey of understanding. And we were all involved in its creation.

Even now, 20 years later, we're still learning the lessons Martin taught us. Sometimes we can hear his voice. *You think the cure for a complicated process like cancer is as easy as stumbling on a gene? Nature is too clever for that—look at how persistent and changeable cancer can be. This isn't like war, with battles shifting boundaries, and winners and losers. This is life.* Sometimes we hear his sardonic laughter when we accept easy answers or lapse into jargon, or we feel his tug on our sleeve just when we think we've mastered some aspect of cancer or let sentiment or wishful thinking cloud our understanding of the needs of people with cancer.

The doctors, as Martin knew and we have discovered, can provide the diagnosis and available biomedical understanding. But all the experts are limited by a particular specialty or by available technology or personal idiosyncrasy. Patients have also been limited by socially and culturally defined roles, as objects to be acted upon, rather than primary actors. Martin helped us to see that we can't accept these limits, that it is up to each of us to enlarge this limited point of view and to encompass and utilize our particular character and skills, our story.

Martin once said that life, art, and science were all the same, just arranged differently. Sometimes everything was dark and confused, especially when you entered a different territory, a territory where death shadowed your steps. Living was the ability to turn on the light and understand whatever was revealed.

Martin died as he had lived, at home, demanding and irritable, amused, clear-eyed about the limitations of conventional care, making use of the complementary therapies that felt right to him, drawing us close for some last observations, a joke about death, a final story.

Now we have far more to offer friends and patients like Martin, new evidence about the power of imagery and meditation, scientific papers on dietary therapies and acupuncture and Chinese herbs, as well as our experience and intuition. We can suggest genuine alternatives for someone like Martin who has run out the string of conventional cancer care and we can nourish hope for an easier and maybe a longer life.

We have a vision now, and the beginnings of a practice of comprehensive cancer care. We also have lessons that Martin taught us, lessons that we have had to learn over and over. We know that survival begins for each of you by accepting and defining the challenge of cancer in your own way. Taking good care of yourself depends on developing a plan of action that looks critically at all the possibilities of cancer care and integrates all the options for treatment—conventional, complementary, and alternative—in a way that is right for you. We know, too, that cancer care requires a team of professionals and the dedication of family and friends. We also know how difficult this task can be.

## About This Book

Mainstream cancer medicine relies on surgery, chemotherapy, and radiation. If cancer is localized, it can be surgically removed and eliminated. Even in cases where complete removal is impossible, surgery, the oldest form of cancer treatment, can be helpful in reducing tumor bulk and controlling symptoms. Radiation and chemotherapy work by killing actively dividing cells. In the process they also destroy normal cells, causing damage to the immune system and side effects, including nausea, vomiting, and hair loss. In spite of the best efforts of well-trained conventional oncologists, over one-half million Americans die of cancer each year.

Recently, some interventions on the genetic and cellular level, including vaccines against cancer, immune therapies, and ways to stop the development of new circulation that supports tumor growth (antiangiogenesis) have been developed. These are only in preliminary trials and are not generally available. They do, however, suggest hope for conventional therapies that are less toxic and more specifically targeted on cancer development.

Complementary and alternative therapies represent another method of fighting cancer. For the most part they are approaches that were not, until very recently, taught in medical schools or used in oncologists' offices or cancer hospitals. Although some, as do conventional therapies, focus on stopping the growth of the cancer cell, many more serve to strengthen the capacity for self-healing of the person who has cancer. They nourish the body's reparative processes, increase its ability to destroy cancer cells, and decrease the tumor burden. They enhance quality of life and help people with cancer to see their illness as more of a challenge and less of a misfortune. These therapies can be alternative to conventional treatment, or they can be used as complements to—together with—conventional therapies.

A truly comprehensive approach to cancer care, the one we are presenting here, is integrative. It uses different combinations of therapies—conventional, complementary, and alternative—in ways that are tailored to each individual patient. As a treatment strategy, integrative care is marked by an openness to different modalities, a willingness to consider whatever works. Integrative care attends to the human being who has the cancer, as well as the cancer he or she has. It emphasizes respectful healing partnerships between physicians and patients. It is grounded in the conviction that, with good information, people with cancer and their physicians can, even in difficult situations, make good choices; that it is possible to create effective, humane, and comprehensive programs of cancer care.

In 1998 the Center for Mind-Body Medicine, a Washington, D.C., nonprofit organization, created an annual conference, "Comprehensive Cancer Care: Integrating Complementary and Alternative Therapies" (CCC). The conference was designed to make information about integrative care available to all those who have cancer and all the physicians, other health professionals, and researchers who care for and hope to help them.

For the first time, CCC brought the researchers and clinicians who had developed the most promising complementary and alternative therapies together with the pillars of the U.S. cancer establishment. Leading clinicians and researchers from Europe, Asia, and Latin America, as well as the United States and Canada, presented their work to scientists from the National Cancer Institute and major U.S. cancer centers. Patients, their families, and their advocates came; so did policy makers and business leaders, senators and representatives. We talked and we listened. Together we began to look critically but open-mindedly at the most promising therapies, to assess how complementary and alternative therapies could best be integrated into care for everyone with cancer.

In 1999 the Center held the conference again, this time with the cosponsorship of the National Cancer Institute and the National Center for Complementary and Alternative Medicine of the National Institutes of Health, and with the collaboration of the American Cancer Society. A third conference, CCC 2000, is scheduled for June 7–11, 2000.

This book is based on those two first conferences. It is grounded in many years of clinical experience with people with cancer and their families and on an ongoing dialogue with those who have done so much to create an integrative approach to cancer.

We have written the book because so many patients, colleagues, and friends have asked us for a reliable guide to complementary and alternative therapies for cancer; because the presentations and discussions at the conferences were thoughtful, authoritative, and useful; and because we believe that the information we are presenting is critical to the care of everyone with cancer.

Our experiences with and perspectives on this enterprise complement each another. James S. Gordon, M.D., is the physician who founded and directs the Center for Mind-Body Medicine. The CCCs were Jim's idea. They are his response to the thousands of questions about complementary and alternative treatments for cancer that had come to him at the Center, as a clinician working in private practice with people with cancer, and in his role as the first chair of the Program Advisory Council of the National Institutes of Health's Office of Alternative Medicine. Together with the Center staff and board, Jim created the CCCs and invited the participants whose work we are here presenting and discussing.

Sharon Curtin is a writer, a patient advocate, an environmental activist, and an expert on the aging process, with a background in nursing and political science. She has learned from her own experience with chronic illness and has long-standing experience helping people with cancer and other debilitating conditions to create programs of integrative care. Sharon and Jim have known each other for many years and have worked together on issues related to health and mental health, particularly of poor children and their families, as well as cancer and other chronic illnesses.

This book begins with an introduction to the experience of cancer and to the terms that describe its diagnosis and treatment. We discuss the shock of diagnosis and present the basic facts you need to know about cancer and research on it ("Facts for Life") and provide a guide to using those facts to your best advantage.

Next we present the most authoritative information about those complementary approaches that offer maximal benefits and may be safely integrated into every person's cancer care: mind-body therapies; nutrition; exercise; group support; acupuncture and Chinese herbs; and above all, an attitude, a spirit of thoughtful and grounded hope. We provide clinical examples—stories—of people who have dealt well with cancer and made complementary and alternative therapies a part of their care.

Much of the information on these alternative and complementary approaches is based on the presentations from the plenary and breakout sessions of CCC I and II, at which papers on research and clinical practice were followed by careful critiques. The benefits and limitations of particular approaches are described, and practical ways to integrate them in daily life are spelled out.

We then provide clear explanations and the most up-to-date, authoritative evaluation of some of the most promising alternative therapies. Until CCC I and II, many of these approaches were ignored or dismissed by conventional cancer care. Some of these approaches, like Dr. Stanislaw Burzynski's "antineoplastons," are medical lightning rods. They have been praised and damned in the national media. Others, like Coley's toxins, Newcastle virus, and Sun's Soup, are little known outside of the cancer underground. Others, like the Gerson diet and Nicholas Gonzalez's program of dietary therapies and detoxification, are widely discussed but seldom carefully considered or thoroughly critiqued by traditional oncologists.

All of these therapies have been selected for this book because they were well presented at CCC I and II by proponents and carefully critiqued by oncologists, and, above all, because they seem to offer very real hope to at least some cancer patients.

We do not have the cure for all cancer. It doesn't exist in conventional biomedicine nor in what has been called alternative medicine. We do know, however, that judicious use of the tools we share with you here and the development of comprehensive cancer care plans can make a difference.

Twenty years ago we didn't have enough good data and evidence to offer Martin the choices we would now recommend. With Jane's understanding and support, Martin charted his own course. He taught us that conventional medical interventions must be judged realistically and skeptically. He insisted that his ability and willingness to experience his life, including his cancer, remain intact throughout the cancer diagnosis, treatment, and his eventual death. Martin was engaged in living his life, by his own standards, every moment. There were limits to his choices, perhaps, but no limits on his ability to be part of what he once called "a grand process—except for the inconvenience."

In this book we offer you the possibility of living life with cancer in a new, expanded, and joyful way, and of making choices that may significantly prolong your life as well as enhance its quality. There are no certainties, but there is certainly another hope entirely.

# 1

# In the Beginning . . .

SARAH FOUND A lump in her breast on May 1, 1995. As usual, she was doing several things at once: taking a shower, planning her day, and performing her regular monthly breast self-examination. Naked, slick with soap, she was thinking about how she could manage to shop for groceries, finish her project at work, and get the kids new sneakers all in that one day. Those few moments alone in the shower were the only time she had for herself; privacy and quiet were associated with the sound of running water, the smell of lavender soap, the smoothness of tile, and the pebbled glass door. When her fingers first found the lump, she hesitated, then probed the spot. She felt her body quiver, as if there had been an earthquake. She immediately thought, *I don't have time for this.*

That moment of discovery was a beginning—and an end. It was the end of her peaceful and lavender-scented sanctuary, the end of her unquestioning and thoughtless confidence in her body. Once she felt this new thing in her breast, the shower became a cold tiled place, where the play of morning light in the water cast a shadow across her skin. She saw her hand groping for a towel and turning off the water. Her hand, her arm, her body, her breast, were suddenly unfamiliar and strange. *I'm not ready,* she thought. *I don't want to begin this, not now.*

Then came the doctors, the diagnostic tests, the biopsies; the search for information, options, resources, trustworthy experts. Sarah sat silently as her body was scanned by mysterious machines and watched as computers talked and technicians said nothing. She stared at the ceiling, naked to the waist, as white-coated strangers felt her breast and discussed her case. She felt vulnerable, as if every time her breast was bared she was being attacked. She tried not to think, not to feel fear. *Don't borrow trouble,* she chanted silently. *Wait until you know.* She smiled, nodded, chatted politely. Inside, she felt herself disappearing, erased and abandoned.

Finally, Sarah sat in her doctor's tasteful office and watched her husband's face turn white with shock as the physician talked about her cancer. She supposed she should comfort her husband, listen carefully to the doctor, ask thoughtful, quiet questions. But all she could think of was how woefully alone and unprepared she was. Panic smothered her, and she sat numb and silent, compelled to hide fear and unable to raise a single issue. It was as if she were only a spectator, standing outside and alone.

Even as she waved away the tissues offered and took her husband's hand, her mind locked on that word. *Cancer.* He said it was *cancer.* The word set loose an echo in her head, a wave of sound crashing against her skull. She reminded herself that she was a competent, practical woman. *I may want to run screaming from the room, and I may resent that I have to think about other people right now,* she thought, *but I have to deal with this.* Finally, the echo faded and she could hear the doctor's voice again.

The doctor, a surgical oncologist recommended by her family physician, spoke slowly, explaining the standard treatment for her stage of breast cancer. Surgery: a simple mastectomy, the removal of the breast and the lymph nodes in her axilla, or armpit, sparing much of the underlying muscle that is lost in a radical mastectomy. Radiation: local, precise radiation to eliminate any remaining cancer cells. Possibly chemotherapy, now or later, depending on what they found during surgery and on how she responded to radiation. Side effects? Minimal and tolerable. They, the cancer experts, would take care of this for her. This is what they knew, this is what must be done.

*What can I do?* Sarah asked.

*Nothing. Just do what we tell you. Our experience shows really good results, and your particular diagnosis suggests a high likelihood of successful treatment.*

Nothing? Sarah felt a gap opening between her and her caregivers. There was their reality—a breast, a lump, a biopsy, the careful scientific studies, the surgeon's experience—and then there was Sarah. The disconnection widened and darkened as the oncologist labored to reassure his patient. He was highly skilled, a recognized expert in breast cancer. Everyone said so. She chose him, believed him to be the best available surgical oncologist.

It was tempting, maybe even easier, to adopt the doctor's viewpoint. He would actively perform and coordinate the best interventions medical science could offer. She just had to cooperate, show up, follow the plan, be a good patient. The oncologist spoke in a flat, cheerful voice that reminded her of high school health classes. He sounded censored, as if confined to some sanitized script. The bad news had the ring of truth, but the reassurances fell flat and false.

Sarah didn't speak of her uneasiness with the proposed treatment or with the way her doctor was talking to her. She wondered if her need for more help and information was something peculiar to her alone. The medical care she would receive would be the best, and she suspected that it was her own weakness that now demanded more.

Until now, Sarah had followed all the guidelines: regular physical examinations, mammograms, self-examination of her breasts each month. She knew early detection and treatment were important factors in successful cancer care, and indeed it seemed that she had found her tumor in a timely manner. Sarah tried to focus on the facts, the numbers, the survival rates, the chances of recurrence, the plans for long-term follow-up care. She noticed her husband's color returning and he began to nod sagely, asking a few questions. *Everyone but the patient felt confident,* she thought.

Sarah was appalled to hear her own voice echo that of her husband's, the quiet and polite response of agreement. *They can always count on that,* she thought. *I respond appropriately, I do the right thing, I defer to the experts, I worry about everyone else and what they think. I want my family unworried, my doctor confident and sure, myself well behaved. This is not a melodrama, not a time for emotional overheating. I am a responsible, stable, intelligent, adult.* She smiled and smiled and felt alone.

Sarah saw the doctor glance at his watch, absently moving her chart to the side. *Well,* she thought. *He's finished, but it doesn't make sense. There must be something I should be doing.* Even as the three of them stood, smiling and shaking hands like people ending a successful business transaction, she made a stubborn and silent vow: *I must shake off the paralyzing numbness I feel—I must find out ways to become active in my own care.*

The decisions were made, the dates for hospital admission and surgery chosen. Sarah held the information packet in one hand and tried not to cling to her husband with the other. *Yes, yes,* she said. *You may as well go to work. I have things to do.* She saw his relief as he turned and moved away with that lanky stride she loved.

Without thinking she moved forward as if to stop him, her empty hand stretching out. As he turned to wave, she clenched her fist into a jaunty gesture, a mocking thumbs-up. *I love you,* he mouthed. *Me too,* she whispered.

*But I won't stick my head into the sand,* Sarah vowed. *There has to be a better way to do this, some way I can connect with my body, my feelings, the people around me. I can't survive feeling so disconnected from an event, a moment as important as this. I've just been told I have cancer, and the news has emptied me out. I have to find a way to deal with the aftershock. The doctors can dismiss my concerns, and my family can expect me to cope with this efficiently. But I know I have to find a way to fill this awful emptiness and overcome the helplessness I'm feeling. I can't do nothing.*

Sarah began her journey in a dark place, feeling alone and ignorant. Surgery, radiation, and possible chemotherapy seemed drastic and mutilating measures, agents of destruction, however necessary. To the doctor, these were ordinary and common procedures. To Sarah, they seemed to be frightening physical invasions that she was forced to endure.

Sarah wanted her physicians to recognize the threat their routine procedures posed to her body, to her. She wanted someone to give her permission to voice and feel her fears, someone to be there for her. She also wanted to discard the passive role encouraged by her doctors, to do something to help herself to feel better while the surgery, radiation, and chemotherapy attacked her tumor. She was desperate for ways to reconnect herself to her body and to her treatment. She remembered reading a book by Norman Cousins, years before, about his experience with a life-threatening illness. Take charge, he advised, in *Anatomy of an Illness*. Be involved, be responsible, do research, find out ways to take care of yourself.

That vague memory was the start Sarah needed. She began what she later called "supermarket research." Determined to overcome her own ignorance, she began gathering information like a student cramming for a final exam. She found books written by cancer survivors. She searched the Internet for information. She read magazine articles and struggled to comprehend professional medical journals. She tried to talk to her family physician about what she was finding out, but found her uninterested or uninformed. Just as the oncologist had dismissed her concerns, her own doctor saw no value in Sarah knowing so much about cancer or in the unconventional, alternative therapies Sarah asked her about.

Sarah felt stupid and even more vulnerable when her questions about acupuncture and herbal therapies to increase her immunity, dietary changes, vitamin and mineral supplements, and relaxation techniques were met with amused glances and dismissive shrugs. None of the doctors was interested in the books she read or the studies she found. *Go ahead and waste your time and money, if it makes you feel better,* they seemed to be saying, *but surgery and radiation is the combination that will work. Science, not magic.*

Still Sarah persisted with her research, feeling she was being driven underground. The specialists worked above, enlightened by science and technology, focusing solely on eradicating the cancer cells. Sarah was in a tunnel by herself, searching for ways to defend and protect and nurture herself, struggling to survive both the cancer and the cancer treatment.

Stubbornly, she began to incorporate some of the information she had gathered into her life. Even though she was initially unsure of the effects of some of the changes in lifestyle she made, it was clear that actively participating in her own care was important—at least to her. It felt as though she were trying to bring light to the dark shadows cast by her diagnosis and treatment. She employed techniques that seemed to help, quit trying to talk about it, and cooperated more or less cheerfully in the conventional treatment plan.

Sarah had a supportive family, her doctor was competent, and her medical insurance coverage was adequate. Five years after diagnosis, she calls herself a cancer survivor. However, she acknowledges that she still struggles with periods of bleak depression and worries about a recurrence of the cancer.

And she is still angry about being treated with condescension, about not being offered good information, and about not being helped to make use of an integrative treatment plan that would maximize her chances for survival and her own peace of mind.

From the time of her diagnosis, throughout her treatment, and afterwards, Sarah needed a guide, a source of information that would provide her with the basic tools she needed to be a partner, an active participant in her healing. She needed a map of an integrative treatment, one that combined the best of conventional oncology with the most reliable and the safest complementary medical approaches. She needed counseling about how to best mobilize her capacity for self-healing and where exactly to find the practitioners who could help her.

When Sarah finally came to talk to us, four years after her diagnosis, we provided support and guidance. We confirmed her hunch that physical exercise and periods of meditation were helpful to her. We worked with her to make sure her diet was designed to help prevent recurrences. We encouraged her to keep on exploring her feelings about the cancer and its treatment with her husband, to make sure they both stayed engaged with her care—and with each other. We referred her to complementary and alternative practitioners who would help and to practices that might make a real difference in how she felt and perhaps, as well, in her chance for long-term survival. Now, in *Comprehensive Cancer Care* we offer this guidance, and those practices and practitioners, to you.

## Coping with Cancer

In her doctor's office, Sarah felt fragile and frustrated, alone and uncertain. She needed far more help than she received. Still, she was soon making use of physical, mental, and emotional resources that would help her through her journey as a cancer patient. She approached her breast cancer as a problem, a natural disaster in her body, that must be understood, directly confronted, and managed. Although it was difficult, she did her best to seek guidance and information that allowed her to develop an integrated, supportive, and active strategy. Of course, not everyone responds to the news of cancer the way Sarah did.

There is, in fact, no "normal" way to respond to the diagnosis of cancer, or for that matter, to any threat or disaster. Numbness, self-pity, bad jokes, physical and emotional collapse, weeping, and outright denial are just some of the immediate defenses that we use. These are responses each of us has developed as protective measures, ways to call "time out" until we are ready to take more direct action. Many of us experience a sort of hyperawareness at such moments: Time seems to slow down or light becomes more intense or we become aware of some small detail with perfect clarity. Sarah, for example, could describe her reaction with total recall four years later. She remembered her tone of voice and even the color of the walls in the room, as she responded to the news of her cancer.

As time goes on our distinctive way of dealing with challenging and threatening situations, of "coping," emerges. Sarah's initial frozen acceptance gave way to determination, her shocked passivity to active engagement in her own care. She overcame her feelings of abandonment and isolation and reached out to her husband and, later, to friends and people who could help her find what she needed. Sarah was prepared, because of her intelligence and personality, to move through shock, assimilate the bad news, and make a personal decision to act. For Sarah, this approach, this way of coping, fueled and energized her search for integrative treatment.

Each of us has a particular way of coping with disaster. All of these responses appear to have certain consequences for our well-being as well as our behavior. And when it comes to cancer, the research suggests that our personal coping styles may have a direct and significant influence on outcome after diagnosis, on how well and how long we live.

Biomedical research has always focused on known and measurable physiological responses to treatment. Beginning in the 1950s, social scientists and psychologists also began to explore the relationship between psychologically determined behavior and cancer outcome. The first studies on coping styles and cancer outcome were influenced by clinicians' observations that some of their patients, with particular characteristics, seemed to do better than others, even if the stage (how early or advanced) and type (breast, prostate, etc.) of cancer were objectively similar.

In several landmark studies, beginning in 1972, Steven Greer and his colleagues in England established a relationship between coping styles and a more favorable outcome for cancer patients. They began by asking whether the psychological stance that patients adopt when they develop cancer can, in some cases, influence the course of their disease. They interviewed a group of women with breast cancer three months after diagnosis and at the beginning of treatment. All of the women had similar diagnoses—a Stage II cancer, which had only spread to some of the surrounding breast tissue—and were treated with surgery and, in some cases, radiation. The researchers discovered that the women's responses could be grouped into four categories:

1. *Fighting spirit:* These patients accepted the diagnosis, adopted an optimistic attitude, and tended to see their cancer as a challenge. They wanted more information and insisted on active involvement in their treatment. These women usually regarded problems as challenges, with solutions that could be found. They were generally energized and motivated toward immediate and active involvement

in finding what would work in any situation. They were natural fighters.

2. *Denial:* These patients either denied or minimized the diagnosis by adopting an attitude of "positive avoidance." They avoided thinking or talking about their cancer and wanted to get on with their lives. Their instinctive reaction was to avoid horrible news or to reduce the impact by concentrating on what they could do. They saw problems as having many layers, not black and white, and preferred to act cautiously and carefully. These women tended to screen information, hearing the part that gave them the best hope. They didn't let the worst news guide their responses. They were not unaware of the truth, they simply gave it less power. These women handled their diagnosis and subsequent treatment by a process of careful denial.

3. *Stoic acceptance:* These women acknowledged their diagnosis but avoided more information. These patients were resigned, fatalistic; they believed there was nothing they could do to help themselves. Indeed, bad things never surprised them. Their strongest characteristic was a stubborn, usually silent, belief in endurance. They rarely complained, or even asked questions. Their coping style was rocklike, stoic acceptance of their fate.

4. *Helplessness, hopelessness:* Their diagnosis completely overwhelmed these patients. They thought of little else and their lives were completely disrupted by their disease. They experienced constant anxiety and did little to improve their mood or general well-being. These women panicked, fretted, and thought in circles. Fear and a belief in their inability to do anything made them both exhausted and ineffectual. They felt sure that nothing in their lives was controllable by them or their actions or needs. They could not conceive of their role as anything but a helpless, hopeless victim.

Greer's study followed patients for 15 years. The psychological response—the coping style of the patient—was related to the disease outcome at 5 years, 10 years, and 15 years. The conclusions are striking. Recurrence-free survival was significantly more common in patients whose coping style was of the fighting spirit or denial varieties than in patients who showed either stoic acceptance or a helplessness/hopelessness response. At the final follow-up, 45 percent of the women who responded to a diagnosis of breast cancer with a fighting spirit or denial were alive and well with no evidence of recurrence, compared with 17 percent who exhibited other responses.

Using similar criteria in other studies, other researchers found that a coping style characterized as either stoic acceptance or helpless/hopeless led to faster progression of cancer in patients with melanoma, cervical cancer, uterine and ovarian cancer, and (in men) the general incidence of cancer. Very recently, a study by Greer's collaborators showed that in another group of women with breast cancer, helpless and hopeless coping styles did have a detrimental effect on survival, but fighting spirit did not seem to improve longevity. Some critics strongly question whether Greer's questionnaire is as valid today as it was in the 1970s, given the vast cultural changes in attitudes that have occurred about illness and cancer. Still, the bulk of these studies suggest that coping style can significantly affect the progression of cancer.

Since coping style is not reaction-specific to cancer, but a pattern and response to threat and trauma learned over a lifetime, is there anything we can do about it, or are we simply to be congratulated or condemned? The answer, fortunately, is that we *can* do something about how we cope. The ways in which we react to crises and cope with them are, in fact, an ongoing process that changes over time, and we have many opportunities to make shifts and transformations along the way. What follows is our outline of the steps you can take in this process. We are describing them for you here so that you can make use of this knowledge to help yourself.

### Step I: Realize That Change Is Possible

Each of us can learn a different coping style. We modify our own clothing and movements in response to weather. We change habits and attitudes and diets all the time, learn new social skills, adjust to new relationships and physical changes as we grow and age. We really do know how to adapt. And once we understand that changing our coping style is likely to improve the quality of our life and perhaps prolong it significantly, we will have plenty of motivation to try to learn to cope differently.

It may seem hard to address the possibility of change, or indeed any action, when one is still reeling from bad news. In fact, however, crisis is mirrored and partnered by change. We know many people, including ourselves, who have made the most profound changes in behavior and attitude precisely when they have been most threatened. "The immediate prospect of being hanged," observed the eighteenth-century English writer, Samuel Johnson, "concentrates the mind wonderfully."

### Step II: Assess How You Actually Do Cope

In the first minutes or hours after diagnosis, and also in the days during which you assimilate and feel the diagnosis reverberate through your thoughts and feelings, you can learn to make an effort to assess how you are coping.

You can start by asking yourself how you have usually reacted to a challenge. What has been your attitude? How have you approached problems and situations that shake your foundations, or events that are disorienting and frightening? It's likely that you'll cope with a cancer diagnosis in much the same way you have been conditioned to react over time. In acknowledging your past patterns, you can begin to modify your behavior.

Sarah felt threatened, alone, and frightened in her oncologist's office. At first she was unable to hear and accept the reassuring words of her doctor or to ask for her husband's support. She was, in short, overwhelmed and numb. Before she could engage in any healing or therapeutic response, she needed time to absorb the news, to survey the frightening new country into which her diagnosis had carried her—"the land of the sick." Then she began to think about how she had dealt with crises before—her parents' illnesses, the loss of relationships—and how she wanted to handle this new crisis.

By the time she drove into her garage a couple of hours later, Sarah's strong ability to actively cope with hardship had begun to banish her fear. She was gearing up, not only to survive the cancer, but to actively seek ways to support and strengthen her body and herself.

The process of assessment is useful for everyone, including those who, like Sarah, obviously possess a strong fighting spirit. Although there are many ways to make this assessment, ranging from the questionnaires that researchers like Greer use, to simply thinking about it as Sarah did, to meeting with a therapist, we have found that the simplest and most direct way is to write down your thoughts and feelings.

Sometimes this process of recording and reflection is at first difficult. Inhibitions about the written word—"Who's going to read it?"—and anxieties about our ability to express ourselves—"Will I get a passing grade?"—often get in the way. It's important to go through this stage, to realize that this writing is for your eyes only, to write down your inhibitions and fears, and to persevere. Sometimes whole pages will pour out, sometimes only a few paragraphs or a few lines. The important thing is to go through this effective exercise.

As you write down your reactions to past and present crises, don't expect, and certainly don't try for, consistency or beautiful writing style. The point is not to create a piece of literature but to discover a part of yourself and your coping pattern. Perhaps you, like Sarah, will put the emphasis on moving ahead and making a plan. Perhaps you will find yourself avoiding writing about cancer, focusing instead on work or family, denying the effects the diagnosis of this disease may have or will have on you. Perhaps you'll notice that you're focusing on the gloomiest possible outcome: If 60 percent of people with your kind of cancer live for 5 years, you may discover through your writing that you are sure you're bound to be among the 40 percent who die sooner. Or you may find that the words you write mirror your overwhelming anxiety, your helpless and hopeless panic.

Whatever your reaction, whatever words, thoughts, feelings, and images, you see on the page, that's where you are right now. And unless you know where you are, it's hard to begin to change, to move on to another place, another mind-set.

Keep in mind that the very act of writing *is* the beginning of change. Psychologist James Pennebaker, and others, have done some wonderful work that demonstrates that writing about a traumatic event—and certainly the diagnosis of cancer is traumatic—has a significant positive effect on the writers' feelings of well-being and, indeed, on their health status and immune function.

These findings dovetail with Greer's research on coping and are of significant importance to people with cancer. Writing itself is an activity, a manifestation of fighting spirit. What you're seeing on the page may be pervaded by the darkness of resigned stoicism or the gloom of helplessness and hopelessness, but the act of writing about it summons the heat of activity and the light of hope. And it may make a very real difference in your physical, as well as your emotional, health.

The first step is realizing that you can change; the second is becoming aware of your coping style. The third step builds on these.

### Step III: Keep Track of What Is Happening in Your Life, Your Mind, and Your Body from Moment to Moment

If you pay attention, you will learn that although you may have a particular "dominant" coping style, you also have other "nondominant" styles. Sarah the fighter sometimes felt helpless and hopeless, sometimes was stoical, and at moments denied what was actually happening to her. This is normal and ultimately reassuring. Becoming aware of these shifts in attitude, particularly for those of us whose coping styles are less effective or productive, reminds us of the reality as well as the possibility of change. Our role is not to force change, but to allow and encourage it to happen.

There are many ways of becoming and staying aware of the manner in which we are coping. Continuing to keep a journal is an excellent one: Write down each day what happened to you and what you think and feel about the day's events. This process provides objective evidence of the process of change and gives us concrete touchstones—words—to which we can return when we feel frightened or lost. It also offers a kind of companionship, a relationship with the words we have put on the page.

Many kinds of meditation (which we discuss in detail in Chapter 3, "Mind-Body Medicine") also provide ongoing awareness of the thoughts, feelings, and sensations that are always arising, always changing in us.

Guided imagery and drawings provide other means for observing our current mechanisms for coping—and, quite literally, for imagining alternatives to them. In the Mind-Body Skills Groups, the support groups of the Center for Mind-Body Medicine, we use an image of an inner guide—an objective version of our unconscious wisdom or intuition—to help people formulate alternative solutions to problems that they confront as they deal with cancer. We also use a series of drawings—for example, of yourself, yourself with your biggest problem, and yourself as you would be without that problem—to help people with cancer explore the challenges that they face and ways of dealing with them.

In the chapters on mind-body approaches and support groups we teach you these exercises. Here, it's important simply to realize that this kind of ongoing self-awareness enables us both to see the changes that are possible and to find and discover specific alternatives to our current coping styles and dilemmas.

### Step IV: Open Yourself to the
### Therapeutic Possibilities You Encounter

As you become more self-aware, or read the remaining chapters in this book, or listen to the thoughts and opinions of those you respect and those who care about you, try to stay open-minded. It was this kind of openness that enabled Jack to join a group and to learn techniques and make connections that were immensely useful to him.

Jack says he survived the Great Depression and World War II by keeping his head down and doing whatever the job required. Like most of his generation, he never started a sentence with "I feel." He was intelligent and aware; he just didn't think about, and certainly never talked about, emotional and personal issues. This was a man who learned early and hard to be tough, strong, a rock. At age 70, when he heard after a regular physical examination by his family doctor that he had colon cancer, Jack faced the tests, the results, the surgery, and the chemotherapy with stoic acceptance.

The struggle showed in his eyes. When he thought about cancer, the deepest pain was never communicated by words, but by a great distance in his faded blue eyes. As far as Jack was concerned, survival was never his to grasp. It was just like the battlefields of Europe. He would live or he wouldn't. He hated talking about his war and his medals, and he hated talking about his colon cancer. Endurance was for him a silent, lonely struggle.

Unfortunately, the coping style that carried Jack through three years of combat was likely to hinder his recovery from cancer. The scientific research that predicts a worse outcome for patients with Jack's stoic personality looks clear and neutral on the page. In real life, it may mean that Jack was risking a dismal outcome because he couldn't complain and wouldn't protest.

Jack certainly didn't consider anything other than the conventional therapy that his doctors offered and didn't even make use of the supportive measures they would have made available: pain control, drugs to treat nausea and vomiting during chemotherapy, nutritional supplementation. He lost too much weight, couldn't sleep, ate very little, and endured pain and constant nausea. He says he just thought that was normal. Fortunately for Jack, his family finally demanded the attention he avoided.

Only after his wife burst into tears and asked him to consider his duty to her and the kids and the grandkids was Jack able to see the value in paying more attention to himself. He was a man who knew about duty. Slowly, his sense of duty allowed him to seek help, encouraged him to learn new survival skills. At his wife's urging, he joined one of the Center for Mind-Body Medicine's support groups. In the group, he became more aware of the silent suffering that only worsened his distress and of techniques of self-awareness, relaxation, and imagery that made him feel more self-reliant and helped decrease the pain. He even came to enjoy sharing his small and large victories with other group members and cheering them on in their own struggles.

By using the same vocabulary and style that put Jack in a precarious position physically and psychologically, his wife was in this case able to help him get out of danger. She appealed to his sense of duty and honor. If Jack had been more self-aware, or his doctors more attentive, this strength could have been recognized earlier and saved Jack considerable pain and complications during the early part of his treatment.

Like Jack, who found the fighting spirit within his habitual pattern of stoicism, all of us have the capacity to open ourselves to change, to become self-aware, to readily mobilize our "nondominant" coping skills and involve ourselves actively in our care. We can develop a new perspective on our treatment and, indeed, our lives.

### Step V: Experiment

Some of the most interesting research on the psychology of health demonstrates the health benefits of taking charge of our own lives and our health care, of looking at the difficulties we face as challenges from which we can grow rather than as disasters that will inevitably overwhelm us. The studies that focus on cancer show improvement in mental attitudes and coping ability in those who begin to explore their emotions and take charge of their own care. The data from more general research on attitude and health are even more impressive and may have significant implications for extending the lives as well as improving the coping style and outlook of people with cancer.

In groundbreaking work Suzanne Kobasa Ouellette, a researcher at New York's City University, found that the people who stay healthy even under significant stress—"the stress-hardy," she calls them—are characterized by a particular set of attitudes. Specifically, they believe they have some control over their lives and exercise it, they are deeply involved in and committed to living those lives, and they take the adverse events that they encounter not as disasters but as challenges. These three factors—which Ouellette calls *control, commitment,* and *challenge*—are the hallmarks of stress hardiness. Like coping styles, these factors can be taught and learned.

Other research also indicates that taking charge may be lifesaving. In their landmark study of nursing home patients, Ellen Langer and Judith Rodin (now at Harvard and Yale, respectively) revealed the therapeutic power of controlling the ordinary events of one's life. Those people who were able to decide what kinds of omelets they ate and which plants were in their rooms not only were happier and more active but also lived significantly longer than those who were simply given—but didn't have the opportunity to *choose*—the same amenities.

There are numerous ways in which you can begin to take control. The approaches and techniques that we discuss throughout this book represent specific healing techniques that you can use—mind-body approaches, nutrition, group support, Chinese medicine, and so forth—to enhance your capacity for psychological and physical self-healing. Equally important, the very act of considering, evaluating, and using these approaches—of acting on your own behalf—enhances their therapeutic potential.

When you no longer consider yourself a victim overwhelmed by cancer, or simply one enduring it, you will be acting on your own behalf, *choosing* the conventional and complementary and alternative approaches that make sense to you. And every time you choose to do this, you are taking control of your life, overcoming helplessness and hopelessness, and transforming your characteristic responses in a life-affirming way.

### Step VI: Create Your Own Integrative Program of Healing

At the end of this book we devote an entire chapter to this process. The important point to recognize here is that an integrative program will be a reflection of who you are, of your unique challenges, perspectives, and needs. The program that you design will probably include many of the approaches and techniques we present in this book as well as conventional cancer care. It will help you in the most concrete ways, physically and emotionally. It will also be the soil from which you grow as a person. Through acting on your own behalf, through caring for yourself, you may well find yourself discovering other possibilities—in every aspect of your life.

### Step VII: Acceptance

An attitude of acceptance begins to grow as, paradoxically, you become active on your own behalf. As you rise to the challenge of surviving cancer, care for yourself, and become aware of what you can control and do, you will grow in understanding. You will recognize and accept what you actually have and what you are doing. And you will realize what you cannot control or do.

The power of acceptance—including a deep acceptance of your cancer—is the shared secret among people who have cancer and other life-threatening illnesses. If we've heard it once in the last 30 years, we've heard it a thousand times: "I would not wish to have had cancer," people of every age, economic condition and race, and diagnostic status say, "but it has been the most crucial, transforming event in my life. Only now," they continue, "have I learned what's really important, who I am, what I can do to really make a difference. Only now that I'm faced with losing everything, do I appreciate everything that I have."

This combination of action and acceptance is a significant part of all the world's spiritual traditions. It is important—and reassuring—to know that possessing this combination, living in its light, may also improve your chances for a significantly longer and more fulfilling life.

## Sarah's Call

Recently, Sarah called and suggested having lunch. She wanted to bring a friend, a woman who was coping with breast cancer, whose experience, Sarah said, was quite different.

Sarah's call was a surprise. Although she had been happy to talk about her breast cancer for this book, not long before she had told us that she felt she had done all that she could about her illness. A few weeks after her diagnosis she had told her husband how overwhelmed and frightened she had been and sometimes still was. He had acknowledged his own fear and how it had kept him from reaching out. Slowly, imperceptibly, their relationship had deepened. They were making more time for one another now, listening a little more. Sarah had also recognized that, as much as her fighting spirit had served her, the experience might have been easier and more fruitful had she relied on her husband earlier and made him more a part of her search and her journey.

Long before she met us, Sarah had moved ahead with her own plan of integrative care, finding help with her diet, a program of physical exercises, and quiet meditation. After she talked with us she felt even calmer and steadier. Her frantic scramble for information and avenues of activity became a strong steady walk. Now, two years after our first meeting, she had decided she wanted to move on. Still, she wanted us to meet her friend, Ann.

Ann was another surprise. First of all, she was older—68 to Sarah's 35—and very shy. Conversation during lunch was slow and sporadic, as if we had met only by chance and were merely being courteous. The two women were clearly fond of each other, and Ann mentioned that she had known Sarah since she was a baby. Because she was a widow, Ann added, Sarah included her in family parties and they spoke nearly every day.

Over coffee, Sarah reported that she was fine, that her last doctor's visit and mammogram showed no cancer recurrence, and that she was, as she had said several months before, ready to stop thinking about the disease. But Ann had been told she had metastatic breast cancer a year ago, and Sarah was helping her through treatment. *I wanted you to meet Ann,* Sarah said, *because she changed the way I think about my experience. Ann handles things differently.*

Ann said little during this conversation, but smiled and nodded and encouraged Sarah like a proud mother. Watching the two women was like seeing generation after generation of women telling secrets, supporting one another, and finding strength together. Sarah said that Ann taught her to value her experience with cancer and to admire her own resiliency. Helping Ann, and telling her what she had learned about breast cancer, sharing her own experience, removed a burden Sarah did not know she carried: a burden of hidden, secret shame about her cancer and her surgery.

*I watched Ann,* Sarah said, *and I saw her going though all this with such dignity and grace. She says she doesn't know why this happened to her, but that it has reminded her of how precious each day is, each person she meets. She has helped me stop blaming myself or looking for reasons where none exist. Ann says that cancer has been, for her, a spiritual experience. She says the cancer provides an opportunity to change, to relearn gratitude, even humility. I wouldn't even know how much I've changed, and how happy I am, if Ann hadn't reminded me.*

And both women did look happy, even joyful. During this conversation they spoke of discovering their bodies as they tried new dietary practices and yoga and meditation. They laughed about how small things were so much more important now—as if the universe had turned up the lights and volume. Cancer, a disease that usually carries a burden of loss and suffering, was expanding their lives. Ann was a devout Catholic, and Sarah, sitting with her in church, had begun to experience a deep peace in her own religious practice.

Ann had been told her cancer was very serious, but this did not seem to preoccupy her thoughts or hinder her activity. Between them, Sarah and Ann supported and simply celebrated where they were and what they were doing. Life was their deepest concern, and finding it joyful, they were happy women.

*The best thing,* Ann said, *is that Sarah is redesigning her bathroom. A new sanctuary, full of light and color. The old efficient tile and shower—gone. Now she'll have a positively sinful Jacuzzi and music and new aromas.*

We were all delighted with the picture. *My own bath,* Sarah sighed. *Where I can hide and plan and soak. And where I will continue to examine my breasts regularly.*

# 2

# Facts for Life

ANYONE CAN DEVELOP cancer, although not everyone does. Still, the numbers are overwhelming. The National Cancer Institute estimates that over 8 million Americans alive today have a history of cancer diagnosis. About 1.25 million new cases will be diagnosed this year, and over half a million of us will die from cancer in 2000. Other than the usually nonfatal skin cancers, the four most common kinds of cancer are breast, prostate, lung, and colorectal. The lifetime risk for the individual—the probability that one of us will develop cancer—is now 1 in 2 for men and 1 in 3 for women. The financial cost of cancer, both to the individual and to society, continues to grow. The American Cancer Society estimates that the annual costs for cancer are now more than $107 billion, more than 10 percent of our entire health care budget.

We know cancer rates have increased because more of us live longer, and cancer occurs more frequently as the body ages; and because screening techniques, which tell us that we have cancer, are more widespread and effective. We also believe, on good evidence, that the way we live and eat, and environmental pollutants—in soil, water, air, and food—are damaging us and predisposing us to cancer. In 1930, the annual rate of cancer mortality in the United States was 143 per 100,000. By 1990, it was 190 per 100,000. Most of the increase derives from the use of tobacco products. In recent years, the deaths of men from lung cancer have decreased. For women, the death rates from lung cancer have increased 147 percent.

We know that preventing cancer is our best defense, and we know that changing behavior reduces the risk of cancer. Some scientists estimate that diet plays a critical role in as many as 40–70 percent of all human cancers and that these could be prevented by the adoption of a low-fat, high-fiber diet. However, if all Americans banished tobacco and fat from their lifestyle, 2 out of every 10 of us would still develop cancer and require treatment.

The facts about cancer are widely available, widely scattered, and susceptible to a wide range of interpretation. Most of us can tell anecdotes or relate isolated statistics or remember a cautionary tale or a promising treatment. Cancer is an ominous and inescapable part of our culture. It is not, however, until we or someone close to us is diagnosed that we must turn our full and fully critical attention to cancer and its treatment.

Cancer is a very complicated disease; in fact, it may be as many as 200 distinct diseases. Mary Ann has a magnet on her refrigerator: "Assume Nothing." She bought it the day she learned she had lung cancer. The diagnosis was unspeakably shocking and, of course, unwelcome, but what made her view life with a more careful and skeptical attitude was what she discovered after the diagnosis—about herself, the disease called cancer, and the medical system. She began a learning process that continues every day she survives her cancer.

*When the doctor told me I had lung cancer,* Mary Ann reports, *we moved right through diagnosis to treatment options. The assumption was that both of us knew what cancer was, or if I didn't, it wasn't important. No doctor I saw ever discussed anything but what was found, and what could be done. I always felt behind, as if I'd come to class too late to learn what I needed to know. It was very depressing.*

Mary Ann, Sarah, and many of the people we see in our offices and meet at our conferences moved from the shock of diagnosis to a realization that they needed to know much more than they were told about their particular cancer. Old or young, scientist, teacher, mechanic, mother, lawyer, doctor, roofer: All felt a need to become an expert on one case of cancer, their own. It was an aspect of their fighting spirit and also a simple commonsense response.

To make wise decisions about the use of various therapeutic interventions, you must make a concerted effort to learn what you need to know. Like Mary Ann, you will probably find out that it doesn't matter how rational and intelligent you are. Fear and ignorance can still lead to bad decisions. Information—and the time to discover whatever you need to know—is one of the most reliable lights in this dark time. Research, asking questions, and insisting on answers are basic good sense actions and may save you money, time, suffering, and even a life.

## What Is Cancer?

There are 10 trillion cells in our body, and we function as living organisms because these cells are generally good citizens. Growing and dividing is the most basic job of the individual cell, and this process is carefully regulated. Too little growth and the body can wither and die. Too much growth and the system is overwhelmed by the malignant, out of control, renegade cells that we call cancer. These cells multiply and spread without control. They crowd normal tissue, stealing energy and nutrition to support their dangerous community. They travel to distant parts of the body, starting new colonies of cancer cells. Eventually, they may threaten the survival of the entire organism.

Biologists and clinicians had developed theories about the nature and function of genes, but until James Watson and Francis Crick discovered the structure of DNA in 1953, no one knew the exact composition and power of the gene. The DNA in the cell's inner portion, or nucleus, it turns out, is structured as a twisting ladder or double helix. This double helix contains millions of subunits, called nucleotides. These units, organized in groups of three, spell out the structure of our genes and create a code that directs the synthesis of proteins in the rest of the cell. This is the master blueprint of all life. Every cell in the body carries this code.

Genes carry information that determines the identity and function of an entire organism and the identity and function of each cell. And each cell in your body carries the code that ordered your brown eyes, your bone structure, and the shape of your body. Tissues and organs develop as the genes organize a process of differentiation and interact with one another according to a precise genetic blueprint. A process of cell division and growth and specialization begins with a single fertilized egg and results in the unique organism that is you. From a flower to a rabbit to yeast to human beings, the process is the same. The genes on the DNA direct the form and function of all life.

Unfortunately, all life forms can develop cancer. The puzzle is why: How could uncontrolled, maverick growth happen? With the discovery of DNA and the technology and tools of molecular biology, science has been able to unlock some of these mysteries, the secrets of abnormal and malignant changes in the DNA and the 100,000 to 140,000 genes that provide our basic operating blueprint.

We now are able to verify what clinicians have long observed: that there are certain families that are predisposed by their genetic makeup to be more susceptible to certain kinds of cancer (for example, families that carry the BRCA-1 and BRCA-2 genes, which are linked to breast cancer). At the same time, we've begun to understand some of the ways that DNA ordinarily repairs genetic damage and to make educated guesses about some of the events that may frustrate repair and lead to cancer.

We've learned that there are genes, carried by each of us in our cells, called "proto-oncogenes" (*proto* is a prefix from the Greek "first" or "before"; *onco* is Greek for "tumor"). Something—cigarette smoke, chemicals, a spontaneous mutation—converts the proto-oncogene into an oncogene, which, acting with other oncogenes, becomes capable of transforming normal cells into malignant cancerous cells.

We've also discovered "tumor suppressor genes" that have the opposite function. Oncogenes, when activated, send signals causing the cell to proliferate, to begin uncontrollable growth and division. Tumor suppressor genes, like the now well-known p53 gene, normally prevent the unregulated growth that is characteristic of cancer cells. If one of these tumor suppressor genes is absent or unable to function properly, then the oncogene is free to act.

The renegade cancer cell is powered by the triggered and active oncogene; its proliferation is facilitated if the usually alert tumor suppressor gene has been damaged. Dr. Robert Weinberg, a research scientist at the Whitehead Institute, describes this as a cell with "the accelerator stuck and the brakes no longer functioning."

Cancer is not a single event with a simple causative agent like a bacterial infection. Scientists believe that cancer arises only after there have been multiple "hits" to different genetic structures, two or usually more insults that convert proto-oncogenes to oncogenes or inhibit the regulatory action of tumor suppressor genes or that disrupt our normal mechanisms of cellular self-regulation and self-repair.

Cancer is also a long and complex drama, a sequence of events unfolding over a considerable period of time, a drama in which customary defenses against uncontrolled cellular division are raised and breached, over and over. We have explained that the DNA has repair mechanisms designed to rectify errors in the genes and to permit the continued growth, development, and replication of normal cells. The body as a whole also has its protective mechanisms, including, most particularly, the immune system's surveillance mechanism, a process in which different kinds of white blood cells can look out for and destroy cancer cells. When cancer cells begin to proliferate they have, in some way or another, overcome these defense mechanisms.

Cancer sometimes has its origin in an inherited vulnerability in the oncogenes or tumor suppressor genes. Sometimes the mutations are created in fetal or adult cells by agents called "carcinogens," cancer producers such as radiation, tobacco use, and toxic chemicals. Sometimes there are other causative agents: hormones and drugs, excesses and deficiencies in diet, or a combination of these.

Once a flaw or mutation exists in our DNA, it may or may not later become cancer. The DNA may repair itself. An oncogene may never be triggered, or an active tumor suppressor gene may do just that: suppress the signal for uncontrolled growth. When the damaged genetic material of a cell escapes these defenses, and the cell is transformed from one that is normal to one that has the potential to create the malignant, uncontrolled growth of cancer, it has entered the first, or *initiation*, phase of cancer.

Once initiation has taken place, the cell is damaged and vulnerable, capable of malignant transformation by communicating and receiving messages spurring uncontrollable cell division. At this point promoters push cells that are damaged, but may not be cancerous, into full rebellion. This second phase is *promotion*. Hormones, such as estrogen, and alcohol, are promoters: They increase the risk of cancer by either triggering or promoting proliferation of cells or by damaging tissue or blocking or slowing the protective action of the body's defenses. Excesses in the diet—for example, large quantities of animal fat—can also be promoters, as can deficiencies of nutrients like selenium.

After mutation and cell promotion, cancer is now present in the body. The conglomeration of cells may remain invisible and silent for many years or the cells may never develop past a very tiny size. Some cancers that are found on autopsy are not the cause of death, but simply rebels who never gained much power.

*Progression* means that the original tumor has reached a point where it causes symptoms (such as bleeding, fatigue, or pain), can be felt (a bump or change in tissue), or can be detected by diagnostic means such as blood tests or an x-ray or imaging technique. By the time a progressed cancer is found, it has doubled approximately 30 times, contains over a billion cells, and has been growing in the body for many months or, indeed, many years.

In early, noninvasive cancers, the growth is confined and limited to one area—as in the phrase "carcinoma in situ"—and has not affected the surrounding tissue. As this primary tumor grows, it needs more room and more nourishment. It begins to develop a supportive circulation and invades surrounding tissues, pushing and crowding. The renegade cell, through multiple steps and influences, has become a mass of malignant cells that are now a destructive and invasive force.

The location of this primary tumor determines its structure and growth: If the normal cells of the affected tissue, like the ones in

Mary Ann's lung cancer, secreted mucous, so, too, will the abnormal cells. One important difference between healthy and cancerous cells is that the cancer cells are less differentiated and fully formed than normal cells; for example, their nuclei, or central portions, may, when you look at them under the microscope, be larger, irregular, distorted. Another difference is that, unlike normal cells, cancer cells do not undergo "apoptosis," or cell death. They just keep on reproducing.

When cancer cells from the original or primary site migrate to distant parts of the body, the progression is called metastasis (from the Greek for "change" or "removal"). If the original or primary tumor is in the prostate or breast, for example, and spreads to the lymph nodes or the bones, it is still a breast or prostate cancer, but one that has metastasized. The type of cancer cells in the metastasis is the same as that of the primary tumor. Like seeds blown far away from the plant, the new tumor will grow and have the characteristics of the original.

Different cancers have different spreading patterns. Breast cancer, for example, tends to spread first via the lymphatic systems to the lymph nodes in the armpit, whereas the cells of other cancers enter the bloodstream and travel to distant organs. Prostate cancer, for example, may be spread via the blood to the bone, lungs, and liver; this pattern is called "hematogenous" spread.

## The Kinds of Cancer

There are three basic kinds of cancer: carcinomas, sarcomas, and lymphomas and leukemias. Carcinomas (from the Greek *karkinoma* or "crab") are by far the most common. They begin in the cells that line the body's internal organs or in those that cover the surface of these organs. Carcinomas include the common tumors of the prostate, breast, lung, and colon. Just like the cells they come from, they may contain secretions of the organs—milk in the breast tumor and mucous in the lung tumor.

Sarcomas come from supporting and connective tissue like bones, blood vessels, and muscles. For example, an "osteosarcoma" is a sarcoma of the bone ("osteo" means bone or bony). Lymphomas, leukemias, and myelomas are cancers of the red and white cells and of the bone marrow and the lymph tissue from which they come.

Within these three general kinds of cancers there are many types, named for the cells from which they originate. A tumor arising from a gland-forming cell in the pancreas would be an adeno (from the Greek for "gland") carcinoma of the pancreas; similarly, a cancer of the flat cells lining the anus would be a squamous (from the Greek for "scale") cell carcinoma of the anus. Tumors are also described by grade and stage as well as type. Low-grade tumors look more like their cells of origin and are not particularly aggressive or invasive. High-grade tumors tend to be fast-growing—quickly invasive—and bear far less resemblance to the cells that gave rise to them.

Cancer staging systems are used to describe how far the cancer has spread and are one factor in determining treatment and prognosis. The most commonly used staging system groups cases into four stages, denoted by the roman numerals I through IV. Stage I cancers are small, localized cancers, whereas Stage IV cancers are usually inoperable and have spread to distant parts of the body. Stage II and III cancers are usually locally advanced and may have infiltrated into nearby lymph nodes.

These stages are defined precisely in different kinds of cancer. The prognosis also depends on the kind of cancer, so that, for example, a Stage II lung cancer has a different prognosis than a Stage II cervical cancer. The system used to more precisely define the cancer is the TNM system: Tumor, Nodes, and Mestastases. Each of these is classified by a number to define the extent of cancer growth. A T1 N1 M0 cancer is small (T1), has one lymph node involvement (N1), and has no metastases (M0). The TNM system is generally used to define Stage I through IV groupings. In his or her diagnosis your doctor may also use other systems, such as the Dukes system of staging the aggressiveness of colon cancer or the Gleason staging of prostate cancer.

## Finding Out What
## You Need to Know

Mary Ann went from being vaguely informed about cancer—from news reports and magazines—to organizing herself as an expert on one case of cancer, her own. From the beginning, she realized that she was confused by what her doctors tried to tell her and that she sometimes hesitated before asking for clarification. She began keeping a notebook. At first it was an anguished list of her concerns and questions as she tried to absorb the news. Soon the notebook grew; she included detailed information on her diagnostic tests, answers her doctor gave, and relevant articles from the newspaper.

Keeping notes was a way of keeping track of all the information Mary Ann had, of questions she had asked and answers she had received. She took it with her to every appointment, with a fresh page filled with new questions to be asked. Mary Ann learned that she had an adenocarcimona of the lung and that it was, so far as her doctors could tell, Stage I.

*I went from panic, through wanting to know why me, and ended up being interested in what was happening. I learned that I needed to be really clear about what I wanted to know, so that I didn't get sidetracked. I had to focus, especially in the doctor's office and when I first tried using my computer to search for information.*

Every bit of information about cancer and its treatment can lead to another, and another. Anyone searching for information on cancer runs the risk of being buried by it. In Appendixes A and B we provide a basic guide to resources to help you with your research. But each of you will have to decide how much information you need, and in what order, to give authority and direction to your choices. For example, Mary Ann began her search with national cancer organizations and found that their information packets gave her the basics to ask more specific questions of her doctor. She also used her computer to correspond with other people with similar cancers. Sarah, on the other hand, read every book she could find written by cancer survivors. She wanted reassurance, and inspiration, before she could move toward more basic clinical information.

Mary Ann did her own research, took notes, asked the hard questions, made the tough decisions, and felt herself grow strong. Although her journey took a different path, Sarah's overall experience was similar. Most often, though, even if your spirit is filled with fight, it's both easier and more effective if you have or find someone else to move with you through the vast sea of information about cancer, the confusion of therapeutic options, and the difficulty and pain of treatment. Clarissa, who came to us for consultation about complementary and alternative therapies, had this kind of partner.

Clarissa, who describes herself as a 45-year-old Washingtonian with "three grown children and two growing too fast," made an appointment at the Center for Mind-Body Medicine after she'd had surgery and radiation and was halfway through chemotherapy for her breast cancer. When asked why she came, she said that she'd heard about the Center from a friend, but that it had really been Ben who pushed her:

*My tough-talking street-smart businessman husband. He took this tumor of mine on as a personal challenge. He came with me to every doctor's appointment. And while I was sitting there open-mouthed and trembling, barely hearing what was said, he asked "why" and "what does it mean" and "what are the statistics" and "could I have copies of the papers" and "who are the world's experts" and "are there other patients we could talk to?" And when we got home, we looked over his notes and discussed everything that happened, and then he got on the phone and the Internet.*

*Sometimes I felt a little sorry for the surgeons and radiologists and oncologists we saw; it was like Ben was doing an audit for a takeover. But Ben learned what we needed to learn—who had done the best work and had the best statistics and whether or not these doctors were willing to answer questions and treat us as if we were intelligent adults. The people who did were the ones we used. And when the time came to look at complementary and alternative therapies—and both Ben and I think we may have been a little late in doing this—I asked some friends and three of them said "the Cen-*

ter." *And we looked up your conference on your Web site. Then Ben made some calls to some of your colleagues to check you out, and here I am.*

Clarissa and Ben exemplify the kind of teamwork we encourage. At the time of her diagnosis Clarissa, like almost everyone, was fearful and vulnerable, ready to simply accept the diagnosis and what was offered to her. If we'd been putting percentages on her coping style we might have called her 50 percent stoic and 25 percent each fighting spirit and helpless-hopeless. But Ben was there for her, involved but not overwhelming, and rarely overwhelmed.

Because Ben was tough, insistent, and attentive to his wife's needs, Clarissa got the information and the help she needed and could concentrate her efforts on getting well. Being there for Clarissa, actively involved, was great for Ben as well. He wasn't a doctor, so he couldn't treat her, but he could use his ability to solve problems, to unearth material that wasn't offered, and to present options and then evaluate them with his wife. In caring for Clarissa, Ben made sure the woman he loved was well cared for by others. When she felt weak after surgery and sick during radiation and chemotherapy, she could relax, knowing he was on watch.

At the Center for Mind-Body Medicine we provide a similar kind of guidance and support for people with cancer. We have focused on the importance of this kind of work in the Comprehensive Cancer Care Conferences, and now we are in the process of developing a national program to train exactly this kind of "integrative care counselor." We believe every hospital and clinic, every oncologist's office, should make this kind of well-informed, impartial but passionate, tough-minded, and tender hearted guide—a Ben—available to everyone with cancer.

Our model begins with an initial one and one-half hour consultation with a physician or other health professional on our staff. We discuss every aspect of cancer and its treatment with the person coming for help, and if he or she wishes, with the family. We give time to the shock and pain of diagnosis. We begin an assessment of coping styles and present the concept of an integrative program. We discuss the ways that conventional and complementary therapies can be combined and assess which ones should be considered and when. And we direct people with cancer to the kinds of resources we list in Appendixes 1 and 2, including the services like CanHelp and CancerDecisions.com that are designed to turn up the latest information on promising complementary and alternative therapies for each particular kind of cancer.

We also offer additional follow-up sessions to discuss the information that has been obtained, to review consultations with other physicians and complementary and alternative practitioners, and to discuss the doubts and hopes that arise. Our aim is to encourage the patient and his or her family to decide what is best for them and to become aware of how each step contributes to or frustrates physical, emotional, and spiritual healing. This book very much reflects this process.

## Mike's Misinformation

Mike left his internist's office feeling worse than he did going in. He had impulsively made an appointment for a physical check-up, vaguely aware he hadn't seen a doctor in a very long time. Forty years old, married, with three children, successful, he was a complacent man with few complaints. His call to the doctor was the act of a man who believed in planning and taking proper care of things: Go to the dentist, clean the furnace filters, check the gutters, take the car in, call your doctor.

Now he wished he had done something irresponsible, like run away to California on a motorcycle, instead.

*He said my prostate was large and my PSA was up and he wanted to biopsy my prostate in six places to see if I had cancer. Nothing was wrong before I went in—how could everything change so fast? I even apologized for wasting his time . . . never met him before and now this problem. Are you sure, I asked him? More tests, second opinion, maybe? He acted like I was a big baby, like I couldn't take the hit. He just kept saying cancer, cancer, cancer.*

Mike talked to his wife and she encouraged him to see another doctor, a urologist recommended by their children's pediatrician.

But before he had that appointment, he began a quest, convinced that science and common sense would eventually prove he didn't have prostate cancer. He felt he was a reasonable man. He would come armed with information, statistics, facts, all proving that he couldn't have cancer. Mike went to his computer, and started a long night staring at the monitor.

He found plenty of information and little reassurance. Plowing through the literature was a bad way to spend an anxious night. Since he had no symptoms and only a vague recollection of the doctor's explanation, he groped and fumbled through various sources of information. *I wanted a big red flash on my screen that said get off—you don't have cancer.*

What he found made Mike lose what little composure he had. He recalls two articles, one on risk factors for prostate cancer, which suggested that he, as an African American, was at high risk for and more likely to develop prostate cancer, and another, a statistical study of long-term survival. Later, he would realize that he misunderstood both pieces of information. Between the dire prediction he thought he heard from the first consultant and the information he saw on the computer, Mike imagined himself in diapers, impotent, incontinent, and then wasting away, gone, and buried. He had all the risks, and the numbers were bad. By the time his wife found him at his desk, crying, he could smell sweet funeral wreaths.

We suspect Mike's experience is not unusual. As a culture we tend to give information and science more weight than understanding. Listening to people struggle with technical information (even professionals who supposedly know how to read research) is a little like hearing someone learn a new language. The most important thing to remember about reading scientific studies or medical news or informational pamphlets is that whatever they say may or may not apply to you. When, for example, scientists discuss "risk factors," it means that the particular quality or behavior or test result they examine may in some measure play a direct role, but not necessarily so. In other words, it does not always contribute to the disease or outcome studied. If you display 9 or 10 "risk factors" for being hit by a car, it doesn't mean you'll ever be hit. You may want to alter the way you cross the street, just in case, but how probability applies in any single case cannot be precisely predicted. Risk is never zero, and seldom 100 percent, either.

With his wife's encouragement, Mike consulted the new urologist. Mike's reportedly elevated PSA (prostate-specific antigen, a substance that all prostate glands secrete) was normal in two follow-up visits. The "enlarged" prostate was large, but, in the opinion of the urologist, within normal limits. And, the doctor added, sometimes PSA levels increase significantly for other reasons—a prostate infection, or even after ejaculation. And besides, Mike learned that only a percentage of men diagnosed with prostate cancer are ever likely to develop a form of the disease serious enough to require treatment or to be fatal.

Mike survived his initial shock and his night of fear, and when he tells this story over dinner, everyone finds it hilarious. He calls it his "how sex and the Internet gave me cancer" story.

As Mike discovered, not all information provides useful knowledge. He came to the conclusion that he was dying based on too little information and poor communication with his first doctor as well as incorrect information, bad reasoning, and a highly developed imagination when searching the Internet. He processed a few facts into a shocking and incorrect understanding. But what if he hadn't been encouraged to seek a second opinion, if he had acted precipitously, if he made a choice for the biopsy based on an incorrect assumption? What if he continued to act as if he had cancer when in fact what he had was a temporarily elevated PSA from having sex with his wife? A biopsy would almost certainly have yielded the same diagnosis but he would have had to continue his journey through the emotional ringer and he would have experienced a painful procedure.

## Choosing Your Medical Team

Mary Ann nodded when she heard Mike's story. Good information, in her experience, is hard to find and evaluate. Yet it is the only guide to making informed choices for everyone concerned with cancer care. Be aware of how much information you want and need. Take your time—seek help, opinions, facts—but try to be open and flexible. Don't assume that any one person, source, or guide has perfect information or expertise. Lasting true statements about something as complicated, and unique, as the treatment of any particular cancer are hard to find. Assume nothing—except, perhaps, a critical and hopeful approach.

This attitude—both critical and hopeful—must inform every step of your journey, including the process of choosing a primary care physician, as well as a surgeon or oncologist. Following are some hints that we've found helpful.

Be sure, first of all, that your physician—or, indeed, any health care professional—is competent. This process should start with the man or woman who is providing primary day-to-day care—your family physician or primary care internist, nurse practitioner, pediatrician, or gynecologist. These people should be appropriately credentialed, preferably "board certified" in their respective specialties. That means they have passed exams in the specialty and have a broad base of both experience and knowledge.

The oncologists, surgeons, and radiologists who may be part of your team should have the same kinds of credentials. It's important, too, to know if they are affiliated with Comprehensive Cancer Centers (ones that have been so named by the National Cancer Institute) or the many more Community Cancer Centers in community hospitals around the country. This affiliation will help ensure a high level of expertise and institutional attention to the diagnosis and treatment of your cancer and the greater likelihood of a team approach to dealing with it.

Those who are offering complementary or alternative care should have—and share with you—their credentials as well. For example, acupuncturists are now licensed in over 30 states and there is a national certifying exam they can take. In Appendix A we provide the names and numbers of some of the national organizations that credential complementary and alternative medicine (CAM) practitioners. And these organizations can, in turn, offer you the names of individual practitioners in your area.

Appropriate credentials are not, however, enough. Mike's first doctor was board certified but, apparently, overly aggressive, insufficiently thoughtful, and unable to communicate clearly. You want somebody who knows who you are, listens carefully to you, and even asks about concerns you haven't yet voiced—a physician who relates to you with consideration and respect. You want a true partner in your health care, not someone who treats you only as a recipient of his or her expert opinions and ministrations.

Your primary care doctor should play an ongoing role in your cancer care. He or she should, we believe, be regarded as your partner, as much a teacher and guide and someone who is responsible for diagnosis and treatment. If you have cancer, he or she should be continually available during your diagnostic tests and treatment, conferring with your specialists, both conventional and complementary, helping you to deal with the consequences of the disease and its treatment, and to make decisions that make sense to you.

All those who are called "caregivers," whether conventional or complementary or alternative, should indeed care. It's part of their job to answer your questions in a way that makes sense to you, to share their rationale for a diagnostic test or treatment plan, to provide data and references that back up their opinions. We tell everyone who comes to us, "If it doesn't make sense to you, it doesn't make sense." The professionals who care for you should meet with your family members, as well as with you, and collaborate with other professionals involved in your care. They should welcome whatever works best for you, not insist on their way.

Many years ago when a dear friend of ours, a 70-year-old physician, had a brain tumor, we went with him to visit three of New York City's most prominent neurosurgeons. Their credentials were impeccable, their neurological examinations equally thorough and elegant. They found the same physical changes, evaluated the lab tests and scans in all but identical ways, and discussed in similar words the possible loss of fine motor function following the surgery.

Their conclusions and the way they related to us were, however, vastly different. Two of the neurosurgeons quoted statistics on the rate of growth of the kind of benign meningioma our friend had and the low mortality (death) and morbidity (disease or damage) from surgery and recommended that we book an operating room. The third neurosurgeon talked with our friend.

Our friend was, himself, a surgeon. His work, so crucial to his identity, so far had been unimpaired by the tumor. This third neurosurgeon did not know any more about possible complications from surgery than the others, but took the time to know our friend and to know that a slight loss of motor functioning might mean a very great loss in his life. He recommended watchful waiting as a treatment rather than surgery.

Our friend worked as a surgeon, unimpaired, for 10 more years, retired, and died 8 years after that—of a heart attack.

## Understanding Terms, Interpreting Data

You need to devote as much time and attention to researching treatment options as you do to finding your healing partners. In the best of all possible worlds your oncologist and your primary care physician will be cordial colleagues and both will be teamed with skilled acupuncturists, herbalists, nutritionists, support group leaders, and yoga teachers. You will have an integrative care counselor, someone trained to help you understand your emotional, as well as physical, needs; to work with you to sift through the research on conventional, complementary, and alternative approaches; and to see which combination is right for you.

This is the model that we are encouraging and creating in the Comprehensive Cancer Care conferences. This is what we hope to train integrative care counselors to do. This is the model of the future. But you, or a loved one, have cancer now. So while we and our colleagues are doing our best to make this model a reality, you need good information and good ways to sort through and understand it. Use the Notes section and Appendixes A and B to access specific books and studies and efficient ways to find information. As you deal with your diagnosis and evaluate treatments, you'll need to navigate safely around the hazards of extravagant claims and fear-producing "facts." To do so, you'll need to understand some of the vocabulary—the terms and statistics—that you'll no doubt encounter.

Mike confused an isolated lab test with reality and leapt from a premature and inappropriate recommendation to a vision of a premature death. Many other people who actually have cancer hear promises of cure in words that only mean modest chances of a longer life.

It seems to us that most people contemplating treatment for cancer want above all to know the answers to two questions: "How much more life is the treatment likely to give me?" and "What will be the quality of that life?" It's important to understand that neither of these questions can be answered precisely, that you are always dealing with some combination of statistics based on averages, the physician's clinical impression, and your own sense of who you are and how what is being recommended fits with what you want for yourself. Still, knowing what the terms mean helps ensure that you'll be speaking the same language as the experts, asking the important questions, and understanding the answers.

*Cure* does not mean that the surgeon has "gotten all of the tumor." Cure means you are likely to live just about as long and as well as if you hadn't had the cancer in the first place.

*Five-year survival*—as in "a 55 to 70 percent 5-year survival rate for surgical treatment of people with Stage II bladder cancer"—means that with that treatment there is a 55 to 70 percent chance that you will be alive after 5 years. Living for 5 years is, therefore, more likely than not, but certainly not guaranteed by these numbers. Moreover, although 5-year survival is a good statistical benchmark, longer-term survival is by no means a guarantee. Some tumors in some people, particularly when they are diagnosed early and slowed down significantly by surgery, radiation, and chemotherapy, still regrow after many years.

*Remission* is a word that is often used, and often confused, with cure. Remission means the "disappearance of the signs and symptoms of cancer" for whatever reason. This means no tumor is visible or detectable and you are feeling no ill effects from the cancer. Remissions can be "temporary" or "permanent"; they can also be "partial," as when some, but not all, of the tumor remains. There are also what are called "spontaneous remissions"—instances when, apparently unrelated to any specific treatment, a tumor disappears. We'll come back to this important but little understood category later in this chapter.

*Response rate* refers to the percentage of people with a particular form of cancer whose tumors are reduced by a particular treatment. Response is thus related to a remission, but not the same as a cure. *Tumor response* means the cancer has changed or responded, in a measurable way, within a designated period of time; it does not necessarily imply an increase in longevity. A "partial response" is essentially the same as a partial remission. "Complete response" means that detectable signs of cancer are no longer apparent, a possible prelude to, although not a certainty of, cure. *Regression* is a related term that refers to a "decrease in the extent or size of cancer."

It's important to pay attention to these definitions, and to the statistics on the percentage of people who experience remissions, responses, and so forth. Treatments are usually recommended based on the studies that produced these numbers, and each of us can use this information to make the best choices for ourselves. It's also important, however, not to be overwhelmed by the numbers. Try not to view them as a predetermined sentence or a ticking clock or a bouncing roulette ball, but as a source of guidance and, whenever possible, an inspiration.

For example, when the Harvard paleontologist Stephen Jay Gould was diagnosed with mesothelioma (a dangerous cancer of the lining of the chest cavity), he discovered research indicating that his prognosis was grim. As he reports, he read the information objectively, both because he is a scientist and because he has "a sanguine nature." He was an optimist in search of information. In his analysis of his chances for long-term survival, he simply decided where in the curve he would fit. If 4 out of 100 diagnosed with his particular cancer survived 5 years, he would be one of the 4. Why not him? The numbers didn't suggest he, in particular, would not survive. They just reported that only 4 percent would, and 4 percent was better than 0 percent, or 2 percent. So he felt pretty good about his chances. And he was right, as it turned out.

## The Evolution of Cancer Therapies and Clinical Trials

Western medicine has been research-oriented since its father, Hippocrates, began to practice and teach on the Greek island of Cos in the fourth century B.C. In the works of Hippocrates we can already see a wonderful balance between research and treatment, between respectful observation of, and experimentation on, nature and a deep appreciation for her mysteries. It was Hippocrates who observed the crablike form of cancer and gave it the name *karkinoma,* which we still use today.

During the Middle Ages, much of Hippocrates's *original* work was lost to Europeans, and with it his experimental methods and expansive spirit. Medieval monk-physicians were scholars, not experimentalists. They learned and parroted the Hippocratic concepts that were passed on to them by Galen of Pergamon, Hippocrates's great systematizing second-century A.D. heir.

The influx of Greek scholars and texts into Western Europe after the Turkish conquest of Constantinople in 1453 revived the emphasis on research. For the first time, Western physicians had direct access to ancient Greek learning. During the Renaissance that followed, classical Hippocratic medicine, like classical art, was reborn. Within a hundred years, Renaissance physicians had planted the seeds for the sciences—anatomy, pharmacology, and physiology—that are still considered "basic" to modern biomedical practice, research, and education.

By the early seventeenth century, the European philosophers Francis Bacon and Rene Descartes were developing a worldview and a scientific method that would foster these disciplines and serve Western medicine's research efforts. Later in the seventeenth century, new technology created new perceptions and possibilities. For example, the use of the microscope opened up a new window on nature: Leeuwenhoek, who developed this marvelous tool, was able to see "animalcules," bacteria that swam in drops of water.

With the invention of more powerful microscopes in the nineteenth century and the careful observations of pathologists like Rudolf Virchow, the focus of medical attention shifted from the organ and tissue to the cell as the basic unit of functioning and of such diseases as cancer. At the same time, the development of increasingly sophisticated diagnostic techniques made possible the delineation of clearer clinical pictures of particular types of cancer and their patterns of spread.

In the mid–nineteenth century, the French chemist Louis Pasteur discovered that specific microorganisms were responsible for particular diseases and developed vaccines against them. The concepts of clear and specific causes, predictable effects, and targeted therapeutics that arose from the "germ theory" shaped a more general model of medical investigation and rational treatment. Disciplined minds making careful observations attempted to isolate cause and effect in cancer.

At the beginning of the twentieth century scientists observed that radioactive substances could cause the cellular changes of cancer. Roentgen, the discoverer of x-rays, and others who used this technology, developed cancers. Soon afterwards, investigators realized that x-rays—which preferentially damage cells that divide rapidly—could also be used to destroy cancer cells.

Meanwhile, the chemical treatment of cancer—chemotherapy—was also evolving. Arsenic-containing compounds had been used from the eighteenth century on to treat cancer. Following World War I, however, it was discovered that mustard gas, which had been used as a weapon, could arrest the growth of malignant tumors. After World War II, Dr. Sidney Farber discovered a compound that inhibited tumor growth by competing with the essential nutrient, folic acid, and soon other chemical substances that selectively attack cancer cells were being discovered and synthesized. By the 1950s radiation and chemotherapy had joined surgery as the accepted treatments for cancer.

Research methodology proceeded from clinical observation to more systematic study. In 1948, the first randomized controlled trial (RCT) in medicine was published in the *British Medical Journal*. A statistician, Austin Bradford Hill, designed the study, which attempted to limit bias by removing subjective judgment and expectations and "randomly" allocating patients to a treatment group and an untreated or "control" group. The disease being studied was tuberculosis, the drug investigated was Streptomycin. The measure of success was survival.

In this study, scientists were endeavoring to remove all influences on survival save one: the antibiotic Streptomycin. Twenty-seven percent of the control group died; only 7 percent of the group receiving Streptomycin died. The researchers also evaluated the chest x-rays of all survivors. The Streptomycin group had more positive evaluations. The study was a success. Streptomycin was determined to be a clinically significant treatment for tuberculosis.

By assigning patients randomly, by "blinding" the study so that neither patients nor doctors know who is getting the treatment (if patients don't know, it is called a "single-blind" study; if neither patients nor doctors know, the study is called "double-blind"), and by carefully following protocols to ensure that patients actually took the appropriate dosage, researchers could point to one drug or treatment as effective or not.

These randomized, controlled, blinded clinical trials are now regarded as the "gold standard," the highest standard of proof in research on cancer. They are designed to demonstrate that a particular new surgical procedure, radiation or chemotherapeutic treatment, dietary change, or mind-body approach has a significant advantage over customary care.

Generally speaking, there are three phases in a sequence of clinical trials. Phase I trials are devised to find out what dose of the treatment is safe and whether there are any signs that it may be effective. Phase II trials are larger and concerned with determining whether and how well a specific cancer responds to the new treatment. Phase III trials are usually, but not always, on a significantly larger scale. They explicitly compare the new treatment with the standard treatment that has been in use. Phase III trials almost always randomly assign patients to either the standard treatment group or the group that is to receive the experimental treatment.

Clinical trials are experiments with "human subjects" and require a careful design and review process by the hospital or other institution where they are conducted. In the United States, most drug studies are RCTs, done under the supervision of the Food and Drug Administration (FDA) and funded by drug companies. They are not, however, the only kinds of valid modern research.

Most medical research starts in the laboratory. To observe the effect of a substance or circumstance, tests are done on cells or tissue (in vitro) or on living animals (in vivo). The experiments are tightly controlled and identical, eliminating chance and as many unknown factors as possible. Sometimes these in vitro and in vivo studies are heralded as major breakthroughs in cancer treatment. There is, however, a great gap between the efficacy demonstrated in the lab, or even in animals, and clinical efficacy in human beings. Humans are very complex physically as well as psychologically, and there are many variables in the way we respond to treatments.

For questions of public health and public policy, long-term observational studies—the work of epidemiology—are crucial. These studies are frequently done to determine "risk factors" that may be associated with or causally related to diseases, like the relationship between cancer and tobacco use or heart disease and exercise. This kind of epidemiological research is often cited in health news stories.

Two kinds of epidemiological studies are particularly relevant: "case-control" and "cohort" studies. In a case-control study, researchers try to compare identifiable factors among groups of people that are similar except for the presence of a disease. In this way, if something is often or always true in the group with the disease, and never or seldom found in the healthy group, a strong relationship is said to exist. How persuasive that relationship is depends on the size and length of the study. In a cohort study, the characteristics and behaviors of large groups of people are evaluated and studied over a long period of time. By using sophisticated statistical techniques, data from these studies can establish important health findings, such as the effects of particular kinds of diet on heart disease or smoking on the incidence of lung cancer.

These are not, however, the only valuable or reliable studies. In recent years a number of new treatments have also been tested in "outcome" studies. In "prospective" outcome studies, the patients who use the new treatment are compared to matched controls who receive the customary care. These studies are not randomized and are not as highly regarded as the gold standard but are, nevertheless, quite useful. So, too, are "retrospective" outcome studies that examine the records of patients who have already been treated by a new approach and compare their outcome to controls.

In recent years the National Cancer Institute (NCI) has encouraged the use of another methodology, the "best case series," as a way to investigate promising new therapies. This approach, which the NCI described in detail at CCC II, asks the investigator to assemble a small number of his or her best cases—8 or 10 or a dozen people—in whom a particular therapy has made a demonstrable and dramatic change, one that would have been extraordinarily unlikely to have occurred by chance.

Best-case series are relatively inexpensive to perform and often obtain results quickly. They are an ideal way to begin to study new approaches, both conventional and alternative, to sort out those that deserve the far more expensive, larger scale outcome studies and clinical trials from those that don't. They also offer the opportunity to study an integrated and individualized approach as well as a specific therapy, like a new drug or herb.

## Scientific Studies and You

If you or a family member already have cancer, epidemiological studies are likely to be of interest. They may give you important hints about some of the "risk" factors—smoking, diet—that may have contributed to your cancer. Some, which we discuss later, may also give you some guidance about steps to take—dietary changes, finding social support—that may help prevent recurrence.

In vitro and in vivo studies are suggestive—it's good to know if a chemical is toxic to cancer cells or if a supplement or herb enhances immunity in a rabbit—but of limited practical value. Clinical trials, outcome studies, and best-case series on a cancer that is like your own are, for the most part, the ones to concentrate on for good information about which therapies may have the most to offer you.

We suggest that you consider asking for and reading yourself the studies of treatments recommended by your surgeon or oncologist or by complementary or alternative care professionals. The studies that are most reliable are those that have been published in scientific, "peer-reviewed" journals. That means they have been reviewed for accuracy, consistency, clarity, appropriate use of statistics, and a host of other factors by scientific peers of the authors/researchers.

Some of these publications seem daunting, with their dense tables and complex tests of statistical significance. Still, almost everyone can understand the abstract or summary at the beginning of each paper and the discussion and conclusions at the end. These are generally pretty clear and make the important points. And you can have some confidence in the accuracy of the material, knowing it has been carefully reviewed.

You may want to ask your physician or a knowledgeable friend about the methodology and the statistical analysis that justify the study's good results. This is particularly important if the treatment has detrimental side effects. You always need to balance potential benefits against possible risks. And we feel it is always useful to have a knowledgeable, fair-minded guide help you in this process.

You may also hear good reports about therapies that have not yet been scientifically evaluated. We suggest you be even more careful in choosing and using them. Above all, you need to make sure that these approaches and techniques will not cause harm or interfere with other treatment. Again, we suggest you review this material with your primary care physician or oncologist.

There is not, however, nearly as much certainty in cancer care as most of us would like. Even when studies are published in peer-reviewed journals and are statistically sound, they are not the last word. Sometimes similar studies have opposing results, and studies and therapeutic practices that are highly regarded at one time may be later discredited. Cancer treatments that were "state-of-the-art" 25 years ago, like the radical mastectomy, are now rarely used. Chemotherapies that are highly touted, and lead to remissions, may or may not actually prolong life. And alternative therapies that appear potent in the laboratory may turn out to be without significant benefit in clinical practice.

It is also important to know that different oncologists (or, indeed, different physicians or alternative care professionals) may select different studies to justify the treatments they use, or interpret and use the same studies in different ways. For example, as Lynn Payer has pointed out in *Medicine and Culture,* American medical and surgical oncologists are far more likely to use aggressive procedures and highly toxic chemotherapies than their equally well-trained European counterparts. It seems to be a matter of the way we Americans think about disease and its treatment, a matter of attitude and temperament, not a matter of the available scientific evidence. Moreover, even within the U.S. cancer establishment, there are wide variations in attitude toward, and use of, conventional surgical, radiation, and chemotherapeutic approaches: Sarah's surgeon was aggressive in performing a simple mastectomy, while his more conservative colleagues would have opted, with equal justification, for a lumpectomy.

## Making Your Choices

Although all these choices may sound—and at times are—complicated and baffling, it is helpful, we believe, to be aware of the complexities and, most particularly, of the need to find solutions that make sense to you. While you're looking at the studies on the effectiveness of particular treatments on your cancer, you always need to assess the effect of these treatments on the rest of you.

We've already noted that some chemotherapies may produce remissions, but not prolong life. Others may prolong the length of your life slightly or significantly but may significantly lower the quality of your life, causing nausea, vomiting, hair loss, weakness, pain, fatigue, and immune system damage. Although complementary therapies are generally nontoxic, there are certainly some alternative therapies that also carry with them significant side effects and inconvenience as well as expense. You need to assess all these factors carefully as you make choices.

We've already mentioned two of the fundamental questions you need to ask yourself as you begin to consider treatment options: "How much more life is it likely to give me?" and "What will be the quality of that life?" Here is a third consideration that will help you evaluate the meaning of the research to you and help you make decisions about your care: What is my life all about? What is my purpose? This may seem a bit far afield or grand, but these are in fact very practical questions.

If you are 35 and your purpose is to stay alive as long as possible to take care of small children, you may want to use aggressive and time-consuming therapies—both conventional and alternative—that offer a real chance at longer life, in exchange for weeks spent in the hospital or at a clinic, months tethered to a demanding protocol, and possibly debilitating side effects. On the other hand, if you are 75 years old and your primary purpose is to enjoy the company of your spouse, visit with your grandchildren, and see parts of the world you've always longed to visit, you may choose a briefer, less-aggressive, less time-consuming approach.

Asking yourself questions about your life's purpose also opens up the possibility of finding that purpose. The diagnosis of cancer and the assessment of your purpose allows you to reconsider what you've been habitually doing and thinking and, indeed, gives this process importance and urgency. For many people—like Sarah's friend Ann—a cancer diagnosis is itself a wake-up call to begin the rewarding process of self-examination and self-discovery.

It's often helpful to do this work with a counselor or therapist—either individually, or together with your family, or in a small group designed for this purpose. Over the years we have seen many people with cancer benefit enormously from this therapeutic process. They are able to identify—often quite rapidly—self-defeating, self-limiting desires, beliefs, and habits, and find new or other ways of thinking, feeling, and living that truly suit and fulfill them.

Finally it's important that you take the time to consider and sift through the possibilities, data, and options—enough time so that when you do make a decision you have confidence in whichever therapeutic approaches you choose. As we suggested above, research data can be read many ways, as can the individual "cost-benefit analysis" of any therapy. A significant study on a therapy you find alien or ridiculous or inappropriate to your life situation is far less likely to convince you to use it than one on a therapy you find immediately congenial. Our experience suggests you should keep an open mind; listen to the experts; find and read the scientific literature; ask for second opinions; take time to talk with friends and advisors; develop a perspective on all the information you have gathered; and finally and most important, make a decision that makes sense to you.

If you use therapies you don't believe in you may well feel anxious, angry, and conflicted every time you go for your chemo or brew your tea of Chinese herbs. These states of mind are almost certainly not conducive to the best possible response. And if the treatment doesn't work as you had hoped, you may blame yourself or feel resentful toward those who encouraged you to undergo it. On the other hand, if you choose an approach that really makes sense to you there are only positive benefits.

In fact, one of the more interesting characteristics of people who survive cancer (and other illnesses) far longer than expected is that they have chosen therapeutic approaches that they believe in strongly, approaches that fit with how they view themselves and the world as well as their cancer. According to many years of work presented at CCC I by Marilyn Schlitz, Ph.D., the research director at the Institute of Noetic Sciences, these people sometimes choose conventional therapy, sometimes alternative, and sometimes an integrative approach. The common denominator of those who experience spontaneous remissions or the remarkable recoveries of unexpected long-term survival is not the technique but the intensity and strength of their belief and the congruence between the kind of approaches they choose and who they are.

Knowing the facts about cancer and its treatment is a powerful beginning. Using these facts in a way that meets your particular needs and serves your unique life purpose gives the facts their true life-giving power.

# 3

# Mind-Body Medicine

TWO YEARS AGO, Tom went in for the regular checkup required by his insurance company. One of the tests revealed occult or microscopic evidence of blood in his stool. Because he was over 50, his doctor scheduled a colonoscopy, a diagnostic procedure allowing the doctor to observe the large intestine. Tom had no symptoms—no pain, abnormal bowel movements, or obvious blood in his stool. He enjoyed good health and wasn't concerned about the test. It was annoying to make time for it in his schedule, and the procedure wasn't something he looked forward to, but he felt no anxiety. He would have the "scope" in the morning and be back at work after lunch. As far as he knew, no one in his family had ever had any kind of cancer.

Three weeks later Tom would discover that just as he was the first in his family to finish college and become a lawyer, now he was the first to be diagnosed with cancer. He was one of about 140,000 people in the United States to be diagnosed with colorectal cancer in 1997, and he was shocked. Tom's doctor was surprised as well, telling him that he had few of the usual risk factors, except possibly age. People with a family history of colorectal cancer have two to three times the risk of an average person. Tom had no family or personal history of polyps, small clumps of tissue protruding from the inner layer of the colon or rectum. He was physically active—he played tennis, skied, and jogged—and usually moderate in his eating and drinking habits. He wasn't a candidate for colorectal cancer but he had it. Now, of course, Tom wanted to know what to do.

Because Tom lived in an area with several good hospitals, includ-ing a major cancer center, he was able to find the kind of top flight surgical oncologist he wanted. He rejected one as too wishy-washy, another as too young and inexperienced, and in the end chose a man very like himself: self-confident, straightforward, and aggres-sive. Both were prosperous from their own labor, and neither one tolerated uncertainty or passivity in their staff or family. They shared a certain cold precision and hot passion for their individual profession—the resolute, fearless surgeon, and the fierce, tenacious litigator.

Tom prepared for surgery believing he had a Stage III cancer be-cause of the size of the growth and the probability of an unknown number of lymph nodes involved. A wide section of his colon would be removed. Because his cancer was aggressive, chemotherapy was planned to follow the surgery. He was told that his 5-year survival chances were 55 to 60 percent or better, depending on the number of lymph nodes involved and his response to chemotherapy. He went into surgery trying to figure out ways to improve his odds.

The surgical results were better than expected: Only one lymph node was involved and the malignant growth was confined to the bowel wall. Tom spent his time recovering from surgery on the tele-phone with clients; using small weights to build upper body strength; refusing to touch hospital food; and basking in the admi-ration of visitors who saw a man in charge, unafraid, in control, and busy with his life.

Chemotherapy was another story; Tom's experience began badly. He suffered from nausea, vomiting, and a terrible headache after the first treatment and both before and after the second treatment. Al-ready impatient with delays in making appointments, he was furi-ous when blood work couldn't be found or the chemotherapy room was overscheduled and he had to wait. He was rapidly losing weight, his color was bad, and he kept imagining his odds getting worse.

*I hated sitting there wondering how I was doing and when I would be treated. I always ended up losing my temper and yelling at somebody, demanding my turn now. By the time I saw the oncologist I would be shaking with rage, weak from hunger, and ready to kill. One day, this technician just looked at me and said I better find a way to calm myself, because nobody got well carrying such a burden of hate and fear and stress. Other people had tried to get me to try diets and prayer and meditation, but this was the first time I believed I would die if I didn't do something else.*

Tom certainly understood stress. For him stress had always been just another part of his life, allowing him to think, act, and respond as required by his profession and the competitive sports he enjoyed. He couldn't function without it. But his colon cancer treatment introduced him to the negative power of stress. He was discovering that his usual responses—his attempts to demand and conquer—were inappropriate and harmful. At first, he had sought more drugs to relieve the tension and anxiety and the nausea and vomiting that came in anticipation of as well as after chemotherapy. But the drugs made him feel like crying or sleeping, side effects he found intolerable. The technician's irritable comment made him realize that he needed new tools to manage this situation, and the helplessness and anxiety he suffered made him willing to act on what he had realized.

Tom believed his will and constitution were strong enough to fight anything, but right now he needed to use his strength and intelligence to find an acceptable way to reduce his anger and anxiety. Nothing in his legal experience, his competitive nature, or his prior understanding of life had prepared him for this crisis. He could fight, but he didn't know how to ask for help, and he certainly had never learned how to relax.

Tom's teenage son suggested he try some relaxation techniques he had learned in a rehabilitation class after a football injury. Tom was dubious, but moved by his son's seriousness and a desire to spare his feelings, he agreed to try relaxing with deep breathing and meditation. His son told him it was like going into "the zone" for athletic activity: All he had to do was concentrate, breathe, and let it happen.

What Tom learned from his son was the practice of sitting quietly and comfortably, concentrating on breathing in and breathing out.

He found lying on the floor more comfortable at first, so he could breathe deeply into the abdomen. As his son led him through the relaxation, he began to feel his body going slack as each set of muscles let go of the constant tension, the constant readiness to fight. He felt as if he were melting into the floor. His son was quiet, one hand on his father's belly encouraging him to continue deep, abdominal breathing.

Tom soon found he could quickly reach a state of relaxation by using deep breathing and hearing his son say, "let the body soften." When he felt distracted, or was interrupted, he learned to bring his attention back to his breathing gently. When his mind started to wander, he let the thoughts come and go and continued the rhythm of the breathing. Twice a day, he practiced relaxation; whenever he needed to calm himself, he took deep breaths and "let the body soften."

Tom was surprised that this exercise required neither faith in its efficacy nor a long period of time. He felt benefits almost immediately—the anticipatory nausea before chemotherapy disappeared and his pain decreased. He was less bothered by delays and less impatient with and angry at everyone. He began to talk with other patients instead of brooding. And, being Tom—a skilled and energetic advocate—he shared his enthusiasm for relaxation, encouraging other patients to try this "little trick."

## Ancient Wisdom, Modern Science

Tom's little trick includes many of the essentials of the mind-body approach to cancer treatment: self-awareness and self-care, relaxation, meditation, and imagery. Tom's response—a decrease in irritation, a quieter mind, a more hopeful attitude toward his treatment, less pain, and fewer side effects—reflects the extraordinary power of this approach and its great promise for people with cancer.

Mind-body approaches—chanting, imagery, hypnosis, and dance, as well as relaxed deep breathing—are as old as the first aboriginal healing systems and as widespread as Chinese, Indian, African,

Latin American, and Native American medicine. It is only in the last 30 years, however, that modern Western medicine has begun to give these techniques the position in health care that they have held elsewhere, the kind of importance they had in the first Western systems of healing in Hippocratic Greece.

Mind-body approaches to healing are based on the understanding that our thoughts and feelings, our beliefs and attitudes, can affect and shape every aspect of our biological functioning. Mind-body approaches also recognize that everything we do with our physical body—what we eat and how we stand, the ways we stretch our muscles and the tension that constricts them—can modify mental and psychological as well as physical functioning. Finally, mind-body approaches are based on the understanding that the mind and body are, in fact, inseparable, that the brain and peripheral nervous system, the endocrine and immune systems, and, indeed, all the organs of the body and all the emotional responses we have, share a common chemical language and are constantly communicating with one another.

In the last 25 years we have learned that mind-body therapies like the one that Tom used can make a significant difference to people with cancer. They offer an opportunity for cancer patients to participate actively in their own care. And, as a rapidly growing body of research tells us, they have the promise to significantly reduce stress and enhance immunity; to enhance the quality of the lives of people with cancer; and, perhaps, even increase the length of their survival.

The scientific frontiers of mind-body medicine were opened in three phases over the last century by pioneering researchers and clinicians who shared a capacity to see and appreciate the power of connections that other investigators had ignored. Walter Bradford Cannon, the great physiologist, paved the way for modern mind-body medicine at the beginning of the century. Cannon, who taught at Harvard, described the dynamic equilibrium, or balance of forces within an organism, as *homeostasis* (from the Greek *homoios*, meaning "similar," and *stasis*, meaning "position"). He also described patterns of behavior and physiology that were common to all the animals he studied, from mice to men. Among these was the response he named "fight-or-flight."

Cannon observed that all animals had a coherent response to a threat, whether the danger was an oncoming storm or a marauding predator. The response included an increase in heart and respiratory rate; greater tension in large muscle groups; coldness and sweatiness; a decrease in intestinal activity; and a dilation, or increase in size, of the pupils of the eyes.

All these, Cannon noted, were manifestations of activity on the part of the sympathetic nervous system, one of two branches of the autonomic ("beyond our control," as opposed to voluntary) nervous system. The sympathetic nervous system, like its complement the parasympathetic nervous system, is regulated in the brain by the hypothalamus. It communicates not only with centers in the lungs, heart, and arteries but also with the medulla, or inner portion of the adrenal gland. There, it provokes the release of epinephrine and norepinephrine, which further stimulate heart and respiratory rate. All of this sympathetic activity, Cannon observed, primes animals—and humans—to flee from a predator or, if necessary, to fight.

The next major contribution to our understanding of the mind-body connection came in the 1920s and 1930s with the work of the Hungarian-born, Canadian physician Hans Selye. As a medical student in the 1920s, Selye had observed that people in the hospital all had a certain "sick" look about them, regardless of their diagnosis. As a researcher, he set himself the task of discovering whether there were consistent anatomical and physiological changes in all these sick people, regardless of the particular illness each endured.

Selye pinched and poked animals and subjected them to heat and cold and loud noises, electrical shocks, and overcrowding. What he learned was that all animals, regardless of the nature of the "noxious stimulus," and in addition to such local manifestations as bruises or burns, showed certain consistent responses. These included an enlargement of the outer part of the adrenal gland, the cortex—which secretes steroid hormones like cortisol that accelerate physiological functioning and decrease inflammation—and shrinkage of the thymus, spleen, and lymph nodes, the major organs

of the immune system. Selye declared that all of these were responses to what he called "stress." He defined stress as "the nonspecific response of the body to any demand" and these physiological changes as "the general adaptation syndrome."

By the early 1970s, researchers were beginning to suggest that the
fight-or-flight and stress responses might contribute to the onset of a
variety of human disease states. According to Cannon's observations, endangered animals quickly flee and quickly recover or else
die fighting. Some "civilized" humans, however, seemed to later researchers to exist in a perpetual state of fight-or-flight. The angry,
time-obsessed, hypertension-and-heart-attack-prone "type A" exec-
utive, described by cardiologists Meyer Friedman and Ray Rosenman, was the prime example. Feeling unable either to fight or flee—
he might lose his job or his status either way—hoping things would
get better, toughing it out, the type A person was in a chronic state
of anxious readiness. In time, Friedman and Rosenman hypothesized, this state produced physical damage, most significantly in the
arteries and heart. Researchers now believe that repressed hostility
is the primary culprit in perpetuating the fight-or-flight response and
in precipitating damage to the heart, but the basic principle—that
prolonged fight-or-flight responses can cause disease—still holds.

Selye's work, on the other hand, suggested a physiological basis
for correlations that were being observed between early or ongoing
emotional trauma—the loss of a parent or a spouse, for example, or
chronic tension—and an increased incidence of cancer, depression,
and other chronic illnesses. Clinicians and researchers suggested
that perhaps people whose immune functioning was compromised
by high levels of stress and prolonged secretion of steroids were
more likely to exhibit both the deficient immune response observed
in cancer and the disordered immune functioning of "autoimmune"
diseases (like rheumatoid arthritis) as well as a vulnerability to
chronic infections.

By the early 1970s it had occurred to many of us that if stressful
situations and stressed-out personalities were conducive to heart
disease, cancer, and other illnesses, it was entirely plausible that decreasing stress and improving outlook might help prevent these ill-

nesses and, indeed, contribute to better treatment. This hypothesis would stimulate new studies on stress-related illness and new ways to deal with it. It would give energy and importance to the new fields of "stress reduction," "mind-body medicine," and "psycho-oncology." And it would, over the following 30 years, provide the impetus for Tom and millions of others around the world to explore a wide range of mind-body therapies.

At about that same time, other lines of research, initiated by George Solomon at Stanford, Robert Ader and David Felten at the University of Rochester, and Candace Pert and Solomon Snyder at Johns Hopkins, were suggesting a third pathway by which mental attitudes and emotional responses could affect physical functioning and produce illness.

In the 1960s, Solomon, a psychiatrist, followed up on a little-known Soviet study that suggested that the hypothalamus is the "headquarters" of immune regulation as well as of autonomic nervous and endocrine system functioning. He found that when he destroyed the hypothalamus in rats, they exhibited a marked decline in immune functioning. Ten years later, Ader discovered that the cells of the immune system, which had always been regarded as an autonomous defense network, could in fact be "conditioned" in much the same way that Pavlov had conditioned dogs to salivate at the sound of a bell. Not long after, Ader's colleague, Felten, demonstrated direct connections between the fibers of the sympathetic nervous system and the organs and cells of the immune system. Meanwhile, Pert and Snyder were revealing that similar receptors for the short-chain proteins called peptides (endorphin is one) exist on the walls of cells in both the brain and the immune system.

Solomon pinpointed the central role of the hypothalamus in immunity. Ader showed that the mind, presumably acting once again through the hypothalamus, could affect immune activity. Felten helped describe the physical connections that make this possible. And Pert and Snyder were suggesting another kind of connection and another mode of communication—peptide messengers—between the cells of the brain and those of the immune system. Ader named the new field they were mapping *psychoneuroimmunology*, to emphasize the interconnections among the mind, brain, and immune system.

As this work accumulated, the connections between the mind and the emotions it produces and three of the body's most important regulatory systems—the autonomic nervous, endocrine, and immune systems—became ever more clear. A panoramic picture of the links among social stress and thoughts, feelings, and physical functioning began to emerge. It looked as if the kinds of stress we experience, and the ways in which we interpret and deal with it, might be significant factors in the production of many of the diseases from which we suffer, as if stress might very well contribute to the onset and course of cancer.

## Stress as a Cause of Cancer: What Do We Know?

For almost 2,000 years, clinicians have observed that people with cancer are more likely to be depressed or grief-stricken, lonely or overwhelmed, than those without the disease—from the second century A.D., when Galen had noted that women with breast cancer were "melancholic," to the end of the nineteenth century, when the distinguished U.S. surgeon, William Parker, observed that "grief is especially associated" with all forms of cancer.

When the psychologist Claus Bahnson reviewed the literature on stress, emotions, and cancer in 1980, he focused on a "particular configuration" in patients with cancer, one "characterized by denial and depression" as well as absence or loss of affection in early childhood, "severe loss" in later life, and strong and persistent feelings of hopelessness and helplessness.

Bahnson had a number of recent studies to draw on: Caroline Thomas's 30-year prospective study of Johns Hopkins medical students, which had revealed a correlation between "lack of closeness to parents" and later occurrence of cancer; Schmale and Spence's observations that women with suspicious cervical cancer biopsies who had recently suffered loss were more likely to subsequently develop cervical cancer; and Le Shan and Worthington's findings that cancer patients were significantly more likely than controls to have "suffered loss of an important relationship" prior to their diagnosis and to "have no ability to express hostile feelings."

In the past 20 years, researchers have sought to confirm these findings and to use the new understanding of psychoneuroimmunology to correlate them with changes in immune functioning. It has become clear, for example, that stress of a variety of kinds—from loss of a spouse to upcoming medical school examinations—can decrease immune functioning, lowering the number of natural killer cells (which seem to be involved in tumor surveillance) and impairing the effectiveness of DNA repair. These findings suggest that stress can make us less capable of defending ourselves against the development of cancer by weakening our defenses against mutations and by rendering immune cells less competent.

More recent studies on personality and cancer have confirmed some, but not all, of the earlier work that Bahnson cited. Indeed, it seems that certain kinds of people are *somewhat* more likely to develop cancer: those who have experienced prolonged stress, particularly stress from which they have been unable to escape; those who have suffered significant losses early in life; and those who have what has been called a "repressive coping" style, a pronounced tendency to deny and repress their own feelings, which has been described as a "Type C personality."

From our point of view, it is useful to know about this work on personality and the incidence of cancer, just as it is useful to know about possible environmental or nutritional factors that may contribute to the development of cancer. It encourages those of us developing programs of cancer prevention—for ourselves and others—to learn to recognize and deal well with the stress we feel, just as research on nutrition helps us make wiser food choices. It is important, however, not to regard these studies as an inevitable prediction of cancer against which we must struggle.

These studies most emphatically do *not* mean that everyone, or even a significant number of people, who has lost a parent at an early age or been under prolonged stress or is uncomfortable expressing feelings will develop cancer. The association—the influence—is, as the gifted researcher Bernard Fox has repeatedly pointed out, at best a *weak* one. And there are many other factors—genetic, environmental, and dietary among them—that probably play far larger roles in the development of cancer.

If you have *already* been diagnosed with cancer, you may be tempted to use this information to blame yourself for some real or imagined psychological failing. When questions arise—"Why me?" or "What could I have done?"—we suggest you pay attention to these questions, but not become preoccupied with them. "Easy to say," many people tell us, "but hard to do." "Yes," we agree, "not so easy but certainly possible." In fact, dealing with these kinds of questions is one situation in which the mind-body approach can be immeasurably useful. If you can relax when the questions arise, they will begin to lose their power to make you anxious and guilty. You can learn from these questions—and from the ways you have previously dealt with stress—instead of blaming yourself or avoiding them. You can see them as a challenge rather than a condemnation, and make good use of them.

For example, there is no definitive way to know whether or not a stressful relationship with a spouse may have contributed to your cancer. There are, however, good ways to deal with this question, this suspicion. You can regard this question as an arrow—guiding you to an area of concern—and deal with the relationship: Make it better, change your attitude toward it, or get a divorce.

If you practice relaxation techniques for a while you will find that it becomes increasingly easy to notice the questions that arise and the answers to them that come to you without obsessing about them so much. Preoccupation with the past is only going to create more stress. In fact, at the most profound level, the mind-body approach is about learning tools to help you let go of the past—with its longings and recriminations—and live comfortably in the present.

## Stress and the Diagnosis of Cancer: Where Do We Go?

A number of studies suggest that stress—and particularly our attitudes toward it—may have far more impact on us after the diagnosis of cancer than before. For example, many studies show that "quality of life"—how someone with cancer feels physically and emotionally, how well he or she functions in the world, and the level of distress from cancer and its treatment—is an important factor in predicting not only how well, but how long someone with cancer will live. That is, if you have lung or breast cancer and you are generally more optimistic and energetic, more involved in your usual activities, and more hopeful about your future, you are more likely to continue to feel better and may, indeed, live longer than if you feel less optimistic or less engaged—even if the type of cancer and its stage are identical.

This research dovetails with Greer and his colleagues' work on coping, and particularly on the destructive effects of hopelessness and helplessness that we discussed in Chapter 1. It is bolstered by studies on the effect of stress on the growth and progression of a variety of different kinds of tumors. Generally speaking, stress—particularly prolonged and major stress (this includes the major stress of life events, such as loss of a job or spouse and, most definitely, of coping both with the knowledge that one has cancer and with its treatments)—stimulates tumor growth. This effect seems to be mediated, in part, by higher levels of cortisol and adrenaline, which depress immune functioning.

This makes intuitive sense. Cancer taxes our capacity to maintain physical homeostasis and emotional equilibrium in many significant ways. It may well make us more vulnerable to situations and stressors with which we previously would have dealt more easily.

On the other hand, knowing that we are vulnerable to stress and what is stressful to us can help us deal with it better. This is true because, ultimately, stress is a subjective experience. If you believe the job you may lose is the only one you will ever have, your level of stress will be vastly different than if you are open to the possibility that losing this particular job may open the door for you to find another, better one. If you see yourself as a helpless victim and cancer as an overwhelming enemy, you will experience far more stress than if you believe you can do something to help yourself heal your cancer and see cancer as an opportunity to find out what really matters in your life—that is, if you see cancer more as a challenge than as a disaster.

The mind-body healing approach is the key to transforming the meaning of cancer and to dealing effectively with the stress it inevitably brings. As soon as you decide to use any of the techniques that are included in this approach, you have already begun to address both your psychological vulnerability to stress and its physiological consequences. Each time you practice any of the techniques we describe below—relaxation, meditation, imagery, hypnosis, self-expression, and exercise—you gain specific physiological benefits: a decrease in stress hormones and enhanced immunity. Each time you feel the benefit of the technique that you are using, you reinforce your sense of control over your own life and counter whatever feelings of hopelessness and helplessness you may feel.

## Relaxation

Relaxation is the most basic of mind-body techniques. It is also our birthright as humans. People in aboriginal or village cultures devote far more time to relaxation than do hyperactive modern men and women. Relaxation is a natural part of their lives, a long pause between activities, and often, as well, the attitude toward all activities they engage in. It is sad but true that most of us in the United States have to make a conscious effort to make relaxation a part of our lives, to remind ourselves of its importance, and to take time for it. When we have cancer we have to make even more of an effort to relax. We need to accept the fear and apprehension that so often accompany a diagnosis and by doing so, soften its impact. Like Tom, we have to begin, in the face of fear and frustration, by *trying* to relax.

Physiologically, relaxation means a reduction in the sympathetic nervous system excitation that marks the fight-or-flight response and a decrease in the level of stress. According to more than 25 years of research, much of it done by Herbert Benson, M.D., and his colleagues at the Mind-Body Medical Institute at Harvard Medical School, relaxation can be powerful medicine: A small quantity can produce significant results. Relaxing 15 or 20 minutes twice a day can lower levels of adrenaline and cortisol; decrease blood pressure, heart rate, and respiration; enhance immune functioning; and balance the activity in the right and left hemispheres of the brain.

Tom's son taught his father a simple relaxation technique; "let the body soften." In our Mind-Body Skills Groups at the Center for Mind-Body Medicine we begin with a similar technique that you can use for yourself: *Close your eyes,* we tell group members,

*breathe deeply, in through the nose and out through the mouth. Imagine your belly is soft. This will deepen the breath and improve the exchange of oxygen, even as it relaxes your muscles. Say to yourself "soft" as you breathe in and "belly" as you breathe out.*

We go on to suggest that our group members—and you—continue this approach for 5 or 10 minutes. Each day you can add another minute or two to it.

*Do this two or three times a day—not right after meals, you may fall asleep—and at bedtime, if you're having trouble sleeping. Use a timer (but not at bedtime) so you won't be preoccupied with how long you've been doing it or how long you have left. Soon, you'll find that in times of stress you can take a few deep breaths and say, "Soft . . . belly," and relaxation will come.*

"Soft belly" is just one of many forms of relaxation. Dr. Benson, who gave a keynote speech at the first Comprehensive Cancer Care conference, has described the almost-infinite variety of techniques that can be used: the repetition of a religious phrase or an ordinary word that is meaningful to you, a prayer or a word like "one," walking or jogging or even quiet repetitive activity. The technique simply needs to be one that is relaxing *for you.*

Regular relaxation has impressive results for people with cancer: decreased levels of stress and increased immune functioning; decreased pain; faster recovery from procedures; fewer side effects from chemotherapy, and less anticipatory nausea and vomiting before chemotherapy; and decreased anxiety, improved mood, and less suppression of emotions. Relaxation also helps you to gain perspective on every aspect of your life and to feel less overwhelmed by it. If you can relax during a difficult time, it becomes, by definition, no longer such a powerful stressor to you. Relaxation is also the basis for the other mind-body therapies and the soil that will nourish their use.

## Meditation

Meditation is a combination of relaxation and self-awareness. Although it is normally thought of as synonymous with a particular technique, meditation is, in fact, an attitude and a way of life, a relaxed awareness of all that arises in our lives and in our minds, of our thoughts, feelings, and sensations. Meditation comes from the same Sanskrit word as medicine and means "to take the measure of" and "to care for."

Meditation is both a technique for bringing us into the present moment and the experience of living in that moment, free from anxiety about the past or apprehension about the future.

There are three basic kinds of meditation. The first, "concentrative" meditation, focuses on a particular phrase or sound (as in the Sanskrit *mantra*, or sound, "Om") or a visual image (a candle or picture). The "soft belly" exercise we just described is a form of concentrative meditation.

The second kind is "awareness" or "mindfulness" meditation. Its prototype is a South Asian Buddhist form called *Vipassana*. In awareness meditation one simply becomes aware of thoughts, feelings, and sensations as they arise. You can do awareness meditation sitting or walking or, indeed, bring awareness to any activity: cooking, cleaning, eating, ordinary office tasks, caring for a child, or making love.

The third form is "expressive" meditation. This includes fast deep breathing, shaking, whirling, and dancing—techniques that move the body and evoke, energize, and release emotions. This is the oldest form of meditation and is still practiced in many tribal societies.

Most of the research that has been done specifically on meditation and cancer has focused on concentrative meditations, which are sometimes described as relaxation and sometimes as meditation. In our experience, however, we have found that all three kinds may be useful for people with cancer, at different times and for different people.

Awareness meditation, particularly walking meditation, is a wonderful way to begin to recognize the rich variety of our thoughts, feelings, and sensations and, watching them come and go, to put them all into a new perspective. By simply noticing our thoughts, feelings, and sensations we gradually free ourselves from obsessing about them. We often suggest that you begin by going outside for 20 minutes and simply walking and noticing the thoughts in your head, the sights of your neighborhood, the smells of trees and flowers, the feeling in your feet as you put one down after the other, the shift in your weight, the swing of your arms, the way you hold your head. It's a wonderful way to become aware of what preoccupies you, to loosen its hold on you as you grow in appreciation of the small wonders of being alive.

Expressive meditation is particularly useful if you're feeling stuck, bogged-down, angry, or depressed. All you need to do is close your door, put on some music, and dance. This is an extremely energizing activity, better done in the morning or afternoon—it may keep you up if you do it before bed—and feels very freeing. Movement brings you into the present moment, allows you to feel energy that illness may have dampened and to enjoy your body, which you may have come to regard with wariness. Sometimes, while dancing, you may find yourself laughing or crying or shouting. Don't push expressive meditation; 5 or 10 minutes to begin with is fine. If you have a physical disability you have to respect its limitations. And, remember, move as your body dictates, not as you think you should move.

If you want to work with a meditation, pick one that is most appealing and set aside a time to do it every day and, if possible, at the same time and the same place. Keep on as long as the technique helps you to move into and enjoy the present moment. If, after a few weeks or a month, you feel it's time to change, do so. You'll learn to trust your own internal compass. If you find yourself stuck and want to ask for help, look in Appendix A for guides. Professionals who have completed the Center for Mind-Body Medicine's training program should be able to help you work with all these kinds of meditations.

## Imagery

Imagery is almost certainly the mind-body technique most widely and happily used by people with cancer—with good reason. Imagery is an innate skill that all of us seem to possess. We all know the pleasure of daydreaming or removing ourselves from an unpleasant situation by letting our mind wander, the exhilaration of imagining things exactly as we want. The practice of guided imagery makes use of this human capacity in a directed and powerfully therapeutic way.

To test the power of images to alter your physical and emotional state, all you need to do is recall the face or voice of someone you love, or breathe deeply and imagine the smell of fresh chocolate cookies, or imagine yourself biting into a wedge of lemon. Notice how your body responds to the images: pleasure and a smile, anticipatory salivation, a puckering of the lips.

In her workshops at the Comprehensive Cancer Care conferences, psychologist Jeanne Achterberg described the basic principles of imagery and its use in cancer treatment. Achterberg, who did some of the first research on the therapeutic effects of imagery with cancer patients, began by defining imagery and describing some of its most striking effects. For Achterberg "imagery is the thought process that evokes and uses the senses, . . . [I]t is the communication mechanism between perception, emotion, and bodily change." Achterberg reminds us that imagery includes auditory, kinesthetic, and gustatory images—those of sound and bodily feeling and taste—as well as visual images. And imagery makes real changes, stimulating the specific areas of our brain as effectively as if we were actually seeing, or hearing, or tasting.

There are two basic kinds of imagery techniques. *Receptive imagery* is the use of a relaxed meditative state to access information from what we sometimes call "the unconscious" or our intuition.

*Active imagery* involves actively imaging some desired result. Both have practical uses for people with cancer.

One receptive imagery technique that we use in all our Mind-Body Skills Groups for cancer patients is the "inner guide technique." The guide is a representation of our inner knowing and our intuition, of the wisdom that can come to us when we are deeply relaxed and paying careful attention. It represents the quiet sureness, unfettered by dogmatism, that exists in each of us. Following is an exercise to help you find and learn from *your* inner guide:

*Sit comfortably or lie down. Begin with a relaxation technique like "soft belly": breathing deeply, relaxing with each breath. Now, begin a journey away from your everyday concerns and the limitations of everyday thoughts, into the realm of your imagination.*

*Imagine yourself walking down a country road. . . . After a while you will notice the sights and sounds and smells as you walk down the road. . . . Pay attention to what you see and feel and hear and smell. . . . After a while you may notice a path that will take you off the road and across a meadow. Follow the path through the meadow, again noticing what you see and feel and hear and smell.*

*After a while longer, you may notice that the path goes through the woods. Follow it through the woods. . . . Perhaps you'll see trees, perhaps flowers, earth, rocks, birds, and animals. . . . There may be a stream off to one side. . . . You may notice, too, that the path goes upward through the woods. Continue and, soon, walking with comfort and pleasure, you'll come to a clearing.*

*Come into the clearing. This clearing is the openness of your imagination, of the space into which intuitive knowing may easily come. Make yourself comfortable. . . .*

*After a while, a person or a creature or a being will appear. It may be a wise old man or a wise old woman, a figure out of mythology, an animal, someone or something you've seen before or someone or something you've never even imagined. This is your inner guide.*

*Introduce yourself to this being and ask him or her or it its name. Know that this being is there to answer whatever questions you have, to help you recover your own inner wisdom. Ask a question.*

*It may be a small question: "What should I have for dinner?" Or it may be something much more important: "What should I do about the pain that I have?" or "How should I deal with a situation at home?" or "What's the best way for me to help myself deal with this cancer?"*

*Accept the answer that comes. Allow it to present itself to you. It may make immediate sense to you, or it may not. It may seem completely accurate. It may be funny. It may just be puzzling. Accept it for what it is. Sit with it. Then, if you would like, ask another question. Again, see what comes. These answers are certainly not the last word on any situation, but they may be extremely helpful in revealing to you aspects of your thinking and feeling that may not have been apparent to you before.*

*After you have your answer or answers, thank your guide, knowing that you can return any time you like to ask more questions. Your inner guide, your intuition, your inner wisdom is always there for you.*

*Begin now, slowly, to retrace your steps. Come out of the comfortable clearing. Walk through the woods. Go over the meadow. Turn back on the country road. And as you walk back on the road, breathing slowly and deeply, you'll find, at a certain point, that it's appropriate to open your eyes and return, finding yourself breathing slowly and deeply in your chair.*

Many people with cancer with whom we've worked find that this process helps them to understand themselves better and to take better care of themselves. The inner guide often serves to remind people of insights and understandings they've forgotten, or of what's really important to them. The inner guide may also help them make decisions when two apparently equally valuable or equally confusing courses of action or treatment are available to them. For example, while Ben—the tough businessman—gathered the facts about breast cancer and analyzed the options, his wife Clarissa used the inner guide imagery to make sure the final choices felt right to her.

Clarissa's inner guide turned out to look a lot like Dopey, one of the dwarves in the movie *Snow White.* Sometimes Dopey answered her questions; sometimes he looked at her in such a sweet, puzzled way that she had to laugh. When Dopey didn't answer right away, the message to Clarissa was clear: Take it easy, laugh at things a little bit more, don't always expect easy answers. At other times, Dopey was more directive. When Clarissa wanted to choose between two oncologists—she and Ben had agreed that both were highly qualified—she asked Dopey. The two oncologists appeared on either side of the dwarf. Dopey looked at each for a while. Then, slowly, he went over to one of the oncologists. He sat in the oncologist's lap and leaned his head against the left side of the oncologist's chest. The message was clear to Clarissa: This is the man with more heart. Clarissa decided to see him and has never regretted her choice.

Active imagery involves the conscious directed use of the imagination to activate a healing response. This is the kind of imagery that was first popularized almost 30 years ago by radiation oncologist Carl Simonton and his wife Stephanie Matthews Simonton. The Simontons encouraged images of immune cells conquering or obliterating cancer cells as, for example, powerful, handsome knights on white horses slaying creepy-looking, ill-equipped armies of cancer cells. In her early studies of the Simontons' work, Jeanne Achterberg showed that people with cancer who spontaneously had these kinds of powerful—even aggressive—images had a better prognosis than those who spontaneously came up with images in which, for example, the cancer cells were overwhelming the white blood cells.

In the years since then, it has become increasingly clear how individualized imagery is. Not everyone wants to or is served by envisioning a battle in which white blood cells destroy cancer cells. The *kinds* of images that are most effective vary from person to person. For example, some people prefer anatomically correct images of white blood cells and cancer cells. Others prefer images that are metaphorical, such as a big broom sweeping up cancer cells. Some people feel empowered by the Simontons' warlike images, but others prefer quieter images: cancer cells fading in smoke or packing up and leaving the body.

Finally, Achterberg describes a third kind of imagery, "end-state imagery." This technique, which is also active, allows you to imagine a successful outcome of an event. While he is still dribbling,

Michael Jordan imagines the ball already in the basket. Cancer patients can use end-state imagery to picture a pain-free diagnostic procedure or a cancer-free body.

Most of the published research on imagery has been on various kinds of active imagery. Indeed, many of the studies combine imagery with relaxation. Sometimes, the studies also compare guided imagery to relaxation. In some studies, the combination of guided imagery *and* relaxation is more effective than relaxation by itself. The effects of relaxation and guided imagery are often hard to tease apart—even "soft belly" is an image. What's important from a practical perspective, however, is that the overwhelming majority of studies show that the combination of relaxation and imagery is helpful for pain control; recovery from cancer surgery; decreasing the nausea and vomiting of chemotherapy; facilitating emotional expression; decreasing the stress response; and increasing the production and functioning of immune cells, including T cells and natural killer cells.

One of Achterberg's research studies—done with music therapist Mark Ryder and published in 1989—suggests that the effects of imagery can be not only powerful but also dazzlingly specific. Achterberg and Ryder found that people could affect different populations of white blood cells depending on which images they chose. Those who imagined one kind of white blood cell, neutrophils, decreasing in numbers, achieved this result while leaving the numbers of lymphocytes intact; conversely, those who aimed to decrease lymphocytes could also do that without affecting the neutrophils. This extraordinary specificity may have important clinical applications for people with cancer, although neither Achterberg nor others who have shown similar changes in immune functioning have been able to make the connection to clinical outcome. It is, in any case, inspiring, a striking example of the way we may be able to use imagery to help ourselves.

## Hypnosis

Hypnosis is defined as a combination of relaxation, suggestibility, and focused attention. It can be understood as a specific way of in-

ducing relaxation and directing guided imagery. Some hypnothera-
pists who work with cancer patients, such as Bernauer Newton,
Ph.D., have emphasized the profound state of relaxation that hypnosis can induce. Newton regards this as the medium in which the
body can restore homeostasis. Others focus on the ways in which
specific hypnotic suggestions may be used, like images, to focus on
decreasing pain or enhancing immune response.

It is very difficult and, ultimately, so far as we're concerned, not
very important to distinguish between hypnosis and imagery. What
is important is that hypnosis, like imagery, makes use of the mind's
extraordinary power to affect physical functioning—or, in other
words, that hypnosis mobilizes the mind that pervades the body.

Research on hypnotic techniques overlaps with, and is at least as
impressive as, the research on imagery. Studies published in peer-reviewed journals have shown that hypnotic techniques can be used
for people with cancer in a variety of ways: to reduce severe pain by
50 percent or more, to decrease anxiety, to improve immune functioning, to diminish the destructiveness of severe burns (from radiation), to decrease nausea and vomiting in people undergoing
chemotherapy, and to facilitate pain-free procedures.

With hypnosis, as well as imagery, it is important that you find
the practitioner—and the approach—that best meet your needs.
Listings in Appendix A are a good place to start, but you'll want to
feel at home with the practitioner as well as confident about his or
her credentials. You should feel deeply relaxed during the process;
satisfied with the guidance being offered and the images that are
suggested; and hopeful about the effect of the technique on your
symptoms, on the course of your illness, and on your attitude toward it.

### Self-Expression

In Chapter 4, "Healing Connections," we discuss at length self-expression in individual therapy and in support groups. Here we
touch on another way to promote emotional expression and self-
help: writing in a journal.

Scientific work in this area is striking. As we mentioned earlier, psychologist James Pennebaker and his colleagues have shown that writing about stressful events—expressing rather than repressing your feelings about them—can enhance well-being, reduce emotional stress, decrease frequency of medical visits, and even improve immune functioning. Published studies have demonstrated the effects of this kind of self-expression in people who have suffered emotional trauma and on patients with rheumatoid arthritis and asthma. There isn't yet any hard evidence of benefits for people with cancer, but we feel the same principles apply. Using this approach clinically, we have seen people decrease their levels of stress, relax more, and feel more comfort in coping with cancer and its treatment.

In the research studies, people are generally asked to write about traumatic events for 20 minutes or more on each of 3 successive days. Cancer and its diagnosis would, of course, qualify as traumatic, and so, too, would any other events that were or are deeply disturbing to you: loss of a parent, a spouse, or a relationship; accidents; terrible disappointments at work; as well as setbacks in your treatment.

We encourage you to spend at least 20 minutes writing on each of the first 3 days and then to *continue* to keep a journal, writing at least a little bit each day, even if only to say, "I don't feel like writing." The focus may be on the ongoing struggles that cancer and its treatment pose, but you may also want to record your thoughts on any and all subjects that seem important to you. Initially, writing about stressful experiences may arouse stress, but over time this exercise significantly diminishes it. We believe that if you make this exercise an ongoing part of your life, it will serve both as a form of self-expression and as a valve for releasing the stress that inevitably arises from the traumatic experiences of cancer diagnosis and treatment.

### Exercise

Physical exercise is often hard for cancer patients to imagine, let alone do. You may feel exhausted from treatment and more frail, older than ever before. The body that once gave you pleasure may now seem like a burden. You may wonder, too, why your oncologist hasn't encouraged you to exercise. These can be obstacles, but they are not insurmountable ones.

Most of us have experienced the results of good exercise: the physical pleasure of movement; the sense, afterwards, of being both relaxed and energized, of feeling at home in our physical body; the heightened feelings of control and mastery; and the improvement in mood that results from increased release of endorphins and other neurotransmitters in the brain. We can recall these benefits, even after a surgical procedure or in the midst of chemotherapy, and remind ourselves that there are appropriate ways for us to experience them again.

In recent years, an enhanced understanding of the psychological and physiological benefits of exercise has encouraged many physicians to make a variety of exercises an integral part of comprehensive cancer care. In place of the fear of exercise that often marked previous eras of cancer treatment, many oncologists are adopting an approach that is shaped by individual self-assessment and by research that shows that exercise can be of significant physical and psychological benefit to people with cancer. It is simply a matter of tailoring the exercise to each person's condition and to his or her likes and dislikes.

Following are some basic principles for exercise:

1. Check on your physical status. Make sure, for example, that you don't have bony metastases, which may make certain kinds of exercise—weight-lifting, contact sports, perhaps even running—hazardous. Make sure, too, that you always consult with your physician about the plan for exercise that you're developing.

2. Find an exercise that suits you *now*. You may have loved skiing before your treatment began, but during chemotherapy, walking may be a much more appropriate form of exercise.

3. Exercise within *your* capacity *now* and push the limits very gently.

4. Include walking as a significant part of your exercise plan. It uses many of the major muscle groups; can give you an aerobic workout; is easy to do; and moves you around, to, and through, pretty and interesting places.

5. Consider experimenting with yoga, *tai chi*, and *qi gong*. These systems of gentle moving meditation—stretching, breathing, and imagery—are an integral part, respectively, of Indian and Chinese medicine. These practices have been demonstrated to have significant effects on increasing muscle relaxation, flexibility, and balance; decreasing pain; increasing depth of respiration; improving mood; decreasing anxiety; and enhancing feelings of well-being and control. Some research on traditional Chinese medicine, which we discuss in Chapter 6, even shows significant improvements in immune functioning among people with cancer who practice *qi gong* regularly.

6. Start where you are. Five or ten minutes of walking or even five or ten minutes of stretching while you are in bed is definitely a beginning. The journey of a thousand miles, as the Chinese proverb says, begins with a single step.

Some last words on the mind-body approach:

1. You need to find the approach or approaches that best suit *you*. We've presented some of the evidence about several of them and shared some of our experiences. The bottom line is that all of these techniques may be helpful for some people and that none of them suits everybody. Find out which ones work for you—and do them.

2. We suggest you use both mental and imaginative *and* active techniques: meditation *and* walking, or guided imagery, journal writing, *and* yoga. Studies have not yet been done on the enhanced benefits for cancer patients of com-

bining these approaches, but it seems pretty obvious that we can only gain by using two approaches that each have benefits, by making the best use of our minds and bodies, and by encouraging all aspects of our being to function optimally and in harmony.

3. Remember that every time you practice one of these approaches, you are not only gaining a specific physiological and psychological benefit, you are also overcoming residual feelings of helplessness and hopelessness; taking control of your own health and your own life; and participating, in the most immediate and palpable way, in your own good care.

# 4

# Healing Connections

WE HIRED THE old mason to rebuild a stone wall. Over a period of years, the forces of water, temperature, gravity, and neglect had scattered the stones in disorderly piles' as if the rocks had been gathered and thrown by a careless hand. No longer a wall, it marked no boundary and offered no protection. The beauty and function of a well-made wall were gone.

The old mason and his helper shuffled the stones and muttered as they worked. *See here—these go together. The wall gets strong by the way these want to connect up. By themselves, these stones have no strength. But put together right, they get strong leaning on each other.*

They worked together in the hot sun, sorting and discarding stones for no reason we could see. But the mason's eyes and hands wove a wall from all those rocks, a structure both strong and beautiful, new and old. We all stood back and admired this creation. Each piece seemed to flow into its fellows, the shades of green and gray as natural and organic as tree bark. We thought of the poet's admonition, "only connect," and added that stonemason's example: Things get stronger leaning together.

We've talked a good deal about the importance of internal or psychological understanding and techniques that influence your experience of cancer and ways to build resources through self-care strategies. Many of these strategies—including analyzing and adapting your coping style and ways of approaching cancer as a life-changing challenge—require working on how you think and react. These skills seem to be based on who you are as freestanding, fully developed human beings who are capable of profound change. We've also discussed the importance of choosing others to help: professionals to diagnose and treat, family and friends to assess options with you, teachers and guides to help you develop your skills with imagery and hypnosis and to create programs of exercise and nutrition that best meet your unique needs.

In fact, the division between self-help and professional care is not so clear. The work of professionals is (or should be) to teach as well as to treat you, to encourage you to care for yourself. And part of self-care is making good choices among treatments and those who offer them. The line between ourselves and others in our lives is similarly blurred. Like the stones in the wall, we gain our identity, our strength, and our function through those to whom we are connected and in the context in which we live. We are the sons and daughters of particular parents; brothers, sisters, fathers, and mothers in specific and unique families; inhabitants of certain neighborhoods, members of an ethnic group, citizens of a particular state; we are employees in this place, employers in that one; now a colleague, now a friend.

There has been a general trend in our Western scientific medicine to ignore this web of connection or to see it as a distant background. In cancer care, the focus is quickly narrowed to the disordered cells, the threatened organs, and the vulnerable body. Most oncologists explore family history only for genetic findings, and address work, if at all, for possible occupational exposures to carcinogens. And all too often those who care for your body actually avoid your psychological issues, social history, and spiritual concerns. If people with cancer, like Sarah, often feel objectified, unknown to their physicians, it is in part because their physicians tend to see them isolated from their rich and complex relationships and from the feelings about these relationships that define them— from the day-to-day social world that shapes, and is shaped by, who they are.

This is not the case in traditional systems of healing. In tribal and village societies, the official healers—shamans, witch doctors, and wise women—who deal with life-threatening illnesses understand that these conditions represent an imbalance in the social order as well as in the body of the affected individual. Healing involves not only herbs and advice but also bringing the extended family or the village together to restore the social balance. These ceremonies purge social dysfunction and reestablish communal connections, the soil out of which all other healing grows.

In recent years we in the industrialized West have slowly begun to recover this wisdom. Increasingly, epidemiological studies and clinical research have helped us to appreciate the power of human connections, and of social context generally, in contributing to, preventing, and treating our most serious illnesses including, most particularly, cancer. Epidemiological studies have informed us that mortality rates are consistently higher among the unmarried than the married and that unmarried, socially isolated individuals have higher rates of infectious diseases, accidents, and suicides. Indeed, one landmark multiyear study of residents of Alameda County, California, revealed that the mortality rates for the most socially isolated men were 2.3 times as great as for those with the most social contacts, and that for women the differential was even greater.

A variety of factors may contribute to these findings—for example, our understanding that poor diet and less regular general health habits are more common among more isolated people. The fact that many, but by no means all, of the data on people with cancer come from studies on women may have some significance as well: Perhaps, in our society, women appreciate and thrive on social connections more than men. Still, the trend is clear: Isolation makes us more vulnerable to cancer; human connections help us to heal.

Recent research has suggested some of the ways in which these kinds of connections work on a biological level. One study on stress in mice showed that the presence of a "mouse friend" decreased the cortisol output in a stressed mouse by 50 percent; when the mouse had 5 friends present, stress no longer produced any elevation of cortisol. The work of Janice Kiecolt-Glaser and her colleagues has not only focused on the power of stress to depress immunity but also on the potency of support groups in mitigating this effect.

The studies on the impact of social support on people who have *already* been diagnosed with cancer are even more dramatic. These studies indicate that people with a variety of cancers who have a higher degree of social involvement—more friends and relatives whom they see, greater participation in religious and other community groups—have a better "quality of life" and, indeed, tend to live longer. One of these studies, by the Canadian epidemiologist Elizabeth Maunsell, was published in the prestigious journal *Cancer* in 1995: Women with breast cancer (confined to the breast or local lymph nodes) who had no confidants had a 7-year survival rate of 56 percent, whereas those with two or more confidants had a survival rate of 76 percent.

## What Kind of Social Support Will Support You?

We have found that the diagnosis of cancer can catalyze both compassion and discrimination. Many people tell us that after their diagnosis they appreciate far more deeply the humanity they share with everyone else on the planet—the vulnerability of our bodies, the swift strokes with which illness may suddenly mark any of us, our common encounter with death. At the same time, cancer makes many people impatient with pointless tasks, the empty forms of some social interactions, and superficial relationships.

This cancer-catalyzed compassion and discrimination can serve you well as you open yourself to those who may want to reach out to you and choose those to whom you will connect. The principles are simple: Reach out to those with whom you feel a connection, to those who understand. Avoid those who dismiss your concerns or distance themselves from you. Do not linger with people who lavish unwanted sympathy on you or swamp you with their own fears. Your cancer will call up everyone's fears of pain and mortality. Those who struggle through their fears toward you can help you to heal; those who run or deny what they are feeling or are overwhelmed by it have a long way to go before they can help. Let them sort out their own issues.

We have discussed the importance of embracing true friends and family and finding proficient professionals who care for your being as well as your body. Here, we want to remind you that the people who use the mind-body approaches we described in Chapter 3 can also be a powerful support to you. But just because someone has more knowledge and is a health professional doesn't mean he or she is going to be helpful. Someone may be a reverend or rabbi or claim to be a spiritual guide, but that person isn't necessarily fit to minister to you. Trust your assessment of these would-be helpers and ask your inner guide for advice. Attending a meditation class with a kind and concerned teacher is an altogether different experience from attending one with a cool perfectionist. The loving hands of one massage therapist feel altogether different from the competent but purely clinical strokes of another.

More formal psychotherapy with a psychiatrist, psychologist, social worker, pastoral counselor, or nurse can also be a wonderfully useful tool. The studies that have been done, and the research presented at the Comprehensive Cancer Care conferences, spell out what common sense tells us. Talking with someone trained to listen, sharing the fears and rage that cancer may bring, listening to someone who will help you learn the lessons cancer has to teach: All these can make a real difference in the quality of your life and how you cope with cancer.

This is not to suggest that everybody who is diagnosed with cancer needs formal psychotherapy. Nor are we recommending the deep probing of the past of psychoanalysis or elaborate attempts to modify behavior. These latter attempts may sometimes actually prevent you from dealing with present issues, frustrate self-expression in the name of behavior change, or obscure your view of the new path that cancer is opening.

Our own experience, our work at the Center for Mind-Body Medicine, and our review of the literature suggest that the counselor's profession is far less important than the way he or she relates to you. Following are some "counselor characteristics" that we've found to be particularly important for people with cancer:

1. He or she is *present* in the sessions, at once alert, thoughtful, and professional enough to help you see yourself in ways you are not yet able to, and intimate enough so that you always feel his or her support and presence.

2. The counselor encourages you to express all your feelings—bad, good, angry, confused, ecstatic, and changing—about the illness, its treatment, and its implications for every aspect of your life.

3. He or she helps you fulfill your own capacity for self-care, assists you in thinking through your therapeutic options, and reminds you always that the choices are *yours*.

4. The counselor is available to meet with your family members and friends to help all of you to see that the emotional pain of cancer may spread to family members even faster than out-of-control cells migrate in the patient's body, that sharing concerns and offering loving support may help to heal all members of the family.

5. He or she understands, as psychologist Lawrence LeShan so eloquently points out, that cancer can be a "turning point" as well a trauma, a time for assessing what is important in your life and even an opportunity for finding new and more meaningful directions.

6. The counselor is flexible. In one recent counseling session with a 40-year-old man with Stage IV colon cancer, we moved from a discussion about the antibiotics used to treat his current infection, to some reflections on why he felt guilty devoting time to himself, to practical instruction in a meditative breathing technique that would help him sleep, to suggestions for talking with his wife about her anxieties rather than trying to solve her problems.

7. The counselor's understanding of the importance of his or her work with you is coupled with an appreciation that this is not the only kind of help available.

8. He or she encourages you to participate in supportive activities other than the one that he or she is offering.

### Supportive Communities and Support Groups

We live in a world that simultaneously frustrates human contact and offers unprecedented opportunities for it. A woman who recently migrated to the United States from Kosovo is appalled at our lack of what she calls "social abilities." So many people she meets are living alone, far from family; everyone seems inordinately busy; no one visits informally, just spontaneously stopping by to talk as the day goes by. There is no *corso*, no evening social stroll, in which a town's or a city's inhabitants daily participate. She finds all this very inorganic and unnatural: How can people develop social relationships when they share so little of ordinary life?

On the other hand, opportunities for connection are as close as the nearest computer and as ubiquitous as the support groups that Americans have created to meet the needs of people challenged by every kind of difficulty and illness. Here again, it is crucial to choose your support wisely and well.

The Internet provides an opportunity for people to share experiences as well as to access information. The quality of the information available is, as you would expect, wildly variable. One of the people who has done the most to use the Internet creatively and sort out the information on cancer care is Steve Dunn. Steve, who has twice presented his work at the Comprehensive Cancer Care conferences, began with a commitment to researching his own cancer and his treatment and in the process changed his life. The more he learned, the more he was moved to share what he knew. In recent years he has embraced the role of supporting others and advocating for better choices in cancer care. His Web site, Cancer Guide, offers an online community for people like him, who are struggling or who have struggled to find the best, the most reliable, information about comprehensive cancer care.

We want to remind you, however, that any Internet sources you find should be reviewed with your caregivers and guides. Equally important, chat rooms and groups are not a substitute for live participation in an in-person support group.

### What About Support Groups?

The history of self-help and mutual support groups in the United States dates back to the beginning of the century. In 1905 Dr. Joseph Pratt organized a program for poor tuberculosis patients in Boston. Working together with recovered patients, he held weekly classes and encouraged those currently with TB to keep a diary. By the 1940s the American Cancer Society was offering places for volunteers to give practical advice and to assist people with cancer in their homes.

In the past 20 years the numbers and types of support groups for people with cancer have grown exponentially. There are groups that provide practical advice—some that deal with chemotherapy and radiation, colostomies and ileostomies—and those that are concerned with spirituality and prayer; groups that are open to anyone with cancer and those confined to people with brain tumors or prostate cancer; groups for adults and for children; large classroom-like drop-in groups whose membership fluctuates significantly from session to session, and closed groups with a fixed membership; groups that meet for a specific period of time, and groups that may go on for years; groups with professional leaders, and those in which the leadership role rotates from patient to patient.

At present, most of the National Cancer Institute–funded comprehensive cancer centers, many community hospitals, and some non–hospital-based oncology practices offer support groups for people with cancer and, on occasion, their family members. There are also organizations that serve more general purposes—like churches, universities, and health clubs—that also offer cancer support groups. There are a number of local programs like New York's Share, which offers self-help for women with breast cancer, and Minneapolis's Pathways, which meets the needs of people with a variety of kinds of cancer as well as other conditions. And there are organizations that began locally but have become national, such as the Wellness Community, which started in Los Angeles, and Gilda's Club (a program of support and education named for comedian Gilda Radner, who died of ovarian cancer), whose first chapter was in New York.

We recognize that different groups meet different people's needs at different times, and we have listed a wide variety in Appendix A. Here, we want to highlight two kinds of group experiences that are particularly powerful and share with you some of the extraordinary research that is being done on them.

## The Power of Small Group Programs

The first kind of support group is small, closed, professionally led, time-limited, intimate, and focused. Stanford University psychiatrist David Spiegel created such a group for women with metastatic breast cancer in 1976. He defined these groups as "supportive/expressive," meaning that the women in them had the opportunity to share with one another what they were feeling and thinking. The groups were led by Dr. Spiegel and other psychiatrists and met once a week for an hour and a half for a year. The women in them learned some relaxation exercises and self-hypnosis to control pain and discomfort. They were also encouraged to talk about what was going on in their lives, in and out of treatment, and about the possibility of death.

The research Spiegel did was carefully controlled. All 86 women received the best conventional medical treatment at Stanford University Hospital. Fifty of them were in support groups, 36 served as controls. Spiegel found that the women in the groups came to care deeply about one another; they helped each other formulate questions for their doctors and sometimes even accompanied one another to appointments. When a group member died, they mourned together.

Spiegel had organized the groups expecting an improvement in the "quality of life" for the women who participated in them. And early results after the last sessions showed that the women were, as predicted, "less anxious and depressed and were coping more effectively with breast cancer." The study was a success and suggested that support groups were an important therapeutic tool.

Ten years after the groups ended, Spiegel did a follow-up study. He was astonished to find that the women in the support groups had lived twice as long as the controls. He doubted his own data, but the finding held and the landmark study "The Effect of Psychosocial Treatment on Survival of Patients with Metastatic Breast Cancer" was published in the distinguished medical journal the *Lancet* in 1989. This was clear evidence that participation in a support group might contribute not only to emotional well-being but also to longevity.

Another study done at UCLA by psychiatrist Fawzy Fawzy and his colleagues confirms that support groups may significantly prolong the lives of cancer patients. In this study patients with melanoma (a potentially deadly form of skin cancer) met with a leader in small groups once a week for an hour and a half—*for only six weeks*. These patients received some education about their disease, learned a few relaxation techniques, did some work on problem solving, were given some "assertiveness training," and had a chance to share their concerns with one another.

Six months after the study ended, the patients in the groups had significantly better natural killer cell activity than those who received only conventional medical treatment. Six years later, group members had a significantly lower rate of tumor recurrence (21 versus 38 percent) and a dramatically lower death rate (9 versus 29 percent).

Finally, a study by Jeanne Richardson of patients with leukemia and lymphoma demonstrated that patients who participated in a modest behavioral and educational home intervention lived significantly longer than those who did not: There was a 39 percent reduction in the rate of death.

Several other studies on other small-group interventions have not confirmed the striking findings of Spiegel, Fawzy, and Richardson. (Interestingly, in two of these "negative" studies there was no significant improvement in psychological status *or* longevity; the patients in the third study had very advanced cancers.) Large-scale attempts to replicate Spiegel's studies in the United States and Canada have not yet been completed. Taken together, however, the findings are impressive, to us and to most of the oncologists we know.

We believe that if you have the opportunity to participate in a group like this and it feels good to you, you should do so. At the very least, you are likely to feel more in control of your life, less anxious and depressed, more hopeful, more connected to other people, and more supported in facing the challenge of cancer. And it is certainly possible that you will be significantly increasing your odds of long-term survival.

The effects of three other small-group interventions that have been presented at Comprehensive Cancer Care conferences have not yet been studied systematically for their effect on survival. They do, however, represent many-faceted variations on the models created by Spiegel, Fawzy, and Richardson, models that in some ways may be richer, perhaps even more hopeful.

These programs, offered at the Center for Mind-Body Medicine in Washington, D.C., Commonweal in Bolinas, California, and the California Pacific Medical Center in San Francisco, emphasize self-care as well as self-expression. In addition, they make considerable use of imagery and meditation, integrate physical techniques such as yoga, and address the spiritual as well as psychological dimensions of cancer.

Commonweal's program is residential and takes place over the course of a week. The others are offered on a regular basis to people from their geographic region. All three programs view the people who come to them as pilgrims in search of healing. All provide enormous latitude for people to explore the purpose and meaning of their lives as well as to develop higher levels of competence in caring for themselves physically and emotionally. All emphasize our connections to one another and honesty and openness in confronting the mysteries of life and death, in addition to better coping with cancer.

## Healing Communities

In recent years successful support group programs have been repli-cated in multiple settings. Commonweal, for example, has orga-nized retreat programs in Hawaii and Maryland as well as in Cali-fornia. And the 500 people who have attended the Center for Mind-Body Medicine's professional training program are currently creating mind-body skills groups similar to the Center's in compre-hensive cancer centers, hospitals, and private practices in the United States and Canada and, indeed, around the world. Information on all these programs is available in Appendix A.

This replication of powerful, effective, and appealing programs only reflects one aspect of an evolutionary process. What began as a unique therapeutic experience—a single retreat or a time-limited group—has begun to evolve into an ongoing healing community. Alumni of Commonweal's retreats meet regularly with one another when they return home. After our 12-week program concludes, many of our cancer groups continue to meet once a month for 2, 3, or even 4 years, to become extended and powerfully supportive families.

At the same time, visionary leaders in other cities have created programs that integrate some of the best aspects of support groups with ongoing classroom offerings in yoga, *tai chi*, and meditation; individual therapies like massage, acupuncture, and energy healing, and practical services like day care. The Wellness Community that Harold Benjamin created in Los Angeles is an excellent example, and has since been replicated in a number of other cities. Gilda's Club provides a similar kind of community, at once social, educa-tional, and supportive. The Center for Attitudinal Healing, which has done some remarkable work, particularly with children with cancer and other life-threatening illnesses, is a third example. These programs—informal, welcoming, and deliberately family-friendly—are supported entirely by donations and are free to all who come.

Recently, Joel Siegel, the movie critic for *Good Morning America* and the national chairman of Gilda's Club, was talking to us about the club atmosphere that had meant—and means—so much to him.

Years ago Siegel's wife had died of cancer, and he himself has re-cently been diagnosed with colon cancer. *As far as I can tell*, he said, *everybody needs pretty much what I need—a place where I can feel comfortable, laughing and crying; people who won't condemn me because I got enraged with my wife for being so sick or look down on me because I sometimes feel so hopeless. All of us with cancer need to be among friends.*

We agree. We feel very strongly that everyone with cancer, and everyone who cares for those with cancer, needs these kinds of groups, these kinds of communities, and this kind of support. The scientific evidence for the effectiveness of support groups—and of strong social networks—is as good as that for many of the chemotherapies that are currently being used. Groups should, we believe, be as integrated into treatment as surgery, radiation, and chemotherapy, as nutrition and the individual mind-body therapies. These groups should also be paid for by medical insurance just as are surgery and chemotherapy.

In Appendix 1 we list ways to get in touch with Commonweal, the Wellness Community, Gilda's Club, the Center for Attitudinal Healing, and other similar organizations to see if there are branches near you. We list local organizations as well. We have a Web site and a phone number (www.cmbm.org; 202-966-7338) where you can find out which professionals have completed the Center for Mind-Body Medicine's training program and who is available in your area.

We suggest, too, that if none of these, or similar, resources are available, you contact your local hospital and insist—politely but very firmly—that it provide these kinds of services. And, in any case, we urge you to start where you are—with friends and neighbors—reaching out so you can receive and give, right now, in your own community.

## Making the Spiritual Connection

One connection that many people with cancer spontaneously find is with something or someone larger than themselves. The name doesn't matter. It could be God, nature, or a "higher power." The connection can be mediated and facilitated by a formal religious or spiritual group or it can be purely individual. In any case, people who feel this kind of connection seem to relax a bit; to feel comforted and supported; and also, interestingly, to become more resilient and self-reliant. Studies on this sense of religious or spiritual connection have shown that having a strong belief system can have a significant positive impact on one's health. The deeper and more profound the connection, the better people's quality of life seems to become.

One aspect of religious or spiritual connections and of support groups that is often neglected is the way in which they encourage us to reach out to help others and the power of this care and concern to heal the person with cancer. It may seem strange that in the midst of the fear of cancer and the pain of treatment you should be encouraged to help others. And yet we have seen, time and again, how energizing and fulfilling this can be. Many people in support groups report that sharing their experience, their deepest selves, touches and reassures others and, at the same time, is powerfully healing for them.

We have known many people whose cancer has helped to spring them from constricting self-involvement to compassion for others, from preoccupation with the most superficial concerns of society to concern for helping the poorest in our society. These are people who have immeasurably enlarged and strengthened their connection to all those around them. But even casual encounters in hospital corridors or on the street can enhance the healing power of connection. Visiting, smiling, offering encouragement, or suggesting small comforts can begin to weave a net of intimacy and social support where none exists.

We suggest you just start from where you are. We all need help and contact and support. And we all need to give help and contact and support. Remember the wall? The stones keep leaning and keep offering strength in their connections. There have been bad storms and fallen trees, and small animals keep making holes here and there, but the wall survives.

# 5

# Diet and Nutrition

WE HAVE TALKED with cancer patients in many settings: mind-body skills groups at the Center for Mind-Body Medicine, consultations in private practice, the CCC, and homes and hospital waiting rooms where we've spent time with friends and relatives who have been diagnosed with cancer. We've consulted with experts, been often to the library, and even taught courses on it. In our experience, no subject has been as promising, or as frustrating, as the role of diet and nutrition in the prevention, and particularly, in the treatment, of cancer.

Over the last few years we've shared some of this information, and its varied interpretations, with many cancer patients individually and in groups. We've been amazed at how much cancer patients—with different diagnoses, stages of disease, prognoses, and treatment status—had to say and ask about cancer and nutrition. Neither social status, severity of disease, nor side effects from treatment seemed to matter. Everyone had questions, confusion, and doubts. And everyone complained that good answers and believable information are hard to find.

In this chapter we present a distillation of what some of the leading authorities have had to say at the CCC, what we feel comfortable and confident in passing on to you. Following is a summary:

- According to two of the world's leading experts, Richard Doll and Richard Peto of Oxford University, as many as 70 percent of all cancers may be related to diet. No one is sure of the exact extent of the contribution of diet. Still, we know that six of the seven most prevalent cancers in the United States—breast, prostate, colon, lung, pancreas, and uterine—show some correlation between cancer risk and dietary factors.

- Although nutritional choices cannot change our genetic make-up, they can directly affect genetic expression, promoting, inhibiting, or masking the effects of genes.

- Obesity is a risk factor for cancer, regardless of the content of one's diet.

- Contaminants in food—pesticides, herbicides, industrial waste, antibiotics, and hormones—as well as artificial flavors, sweeteners, and colorings may play a role in cancer promotion.

- Scientific research that addresses the relationship between diet and cancer, including thousands of careful studies, is available to patients and clinicians.

- Cancer patients have demonstrated a willingness to make significant dietary changes when given compelling evidence.

- Most oncologists and other physicians have been poorly prepared either to give basic, good nutritional information or to advise patients on specific nutritional strategies for treatment and prevention.

- Everyone has to eat, every day. Once the correlation between dietary factors and every stage of cancer is understood, nutritional strategies become an obvious and easy therapeutic intervention.

- Even when our scientific data are incomplete, we must, as doctors and patients, act on the best available evidence-based information.

- Although the recommendations we make are based on the best available evidence, it is important to understand that there are significant biochemical differences among us—that no one diet will be right for everyone with cancer.

Based on our understanding of the available data, we believe that all cancer patients will benefit from the following general guidelines, which are detailed and discussed in this chapter:

- Eat a low-fat, high-fiber diet based primarily on vegetables, fruits, and whole grains.
- Eat less red meat and more fish or skinless chicken.
- Include essential fatty acids, fish oils (from supplements or deep-water fish), and olive oil. Avoid other vegetable oils, particularly hydrogenated oils such as margarine.
- Include specific foods with known anticancer action, including cruciferous vegetables (broccoli, cabbage, brussels sprouts), soy products, and berries.
- Eat more fresh and whole foods, particularly avoiding processed food and food to which colorings, preservatives, and other chemicals have been added.
- Eat organic foods if you can find, and afford, them.
- Pay attention to the way foods affect you. We all respond differently to food, have different needs and sensitivities.
- Add supplements to your regular routine, including antioxidant vitamins and selenium.
- Eat slowly, tasting and enjoying what you eat.
- Report dietary changes and any supplements you take to the health professionals involved in your care. Discuss all aspects of nutrition with them. Nutrition is part of your care. They should be interested, and should be, or should become, knowledgeable.

## You Are What You Eat

Nutritional habits are developed over a lifetime of eating. Where you grew up and your family background—including regional differences and ethnic influences—help to form the basis of personal preference. If you grew up in the southern United States, you probably prefer rice as the main starch in your diet; in the North, people eat more potatoes. Food choice is affected by advertising and marketing, by availability and price. The skill and preferences of whoever cooked for you as a child also influence early development of taste, flexibility, and identification of "comfort foods." Individual taste, even within families, varies significantly.

Concern about the shape of our bodies, as well as questions about diet and health, fuels a search for the "best diet." Diet books fly out of bookstores. Popular books on nutrition often offer "evidence-based" advice and promise therapeutic changes. There is usually some truth in all these books, whether they focus on increasing insulin efficiency or lowering cholesterol or weight loss or cancer prevention. There may be scientific data supporting the book's basic premise or plausible anecdotal evidence. The books, however, contradict one another, often quite vehemently.

Ordinarily readers embrace one set of dietary solutions, cleave to it if it seems to work, drop it if doesn't, and move on to the next possible answer. For people with cancer the stakes are higher and the distress greater. At a time of great vulnerability, people must choose among what appear to be contradictory recommendations. In a time of fear, it often seems they must make profound changes in one of the reassuring constants in their life—their food.

Over the years we have learned that all people, but especially those with cancer, want and need simple guidelines, backed by authority. They want access to scientific data and explanations of the biochemistry and action of nutrients to support their decisions. We have found that this kind of information gives people with cancer the most flexibility and helps to inspire necessary changes. At the same time, almost everyone with cancer we know has reported a lack of guidance from doctors. Few felt they had received useful information from their oncologists or other health care providers, even when they specifically asked for it.

What were they told?: "Follow a healthy diet," or "Keep your weight stable," or "Eat enough of whatever you like," or, at best— and it is definitely better—"Eat more fruits and vegetables." The more honest answer, more than one patient has suggested, would have been for doctors to say they don't know.

Over the years we've found, as we do give specific nutritional information to patients, that some are significantly more reluctant to accept it—and to change—than others. We met Don because his wife persuaded him that he needed to do something about his diet. He was almost 60 years old, about 30 pounds overweight, and his union required an employer-paid yearly physical, including a colonoscopy (examination of the large bowel with a flexible tube equipped with a "scope"). The year we met him, a malignant tumor was found in his colon through this screening. His wife believed job stress and bad food—"too much fast food and grease"—contributed to the development of his cancer.

Don, on the other hand, liked his high-pressure job and liked the food his wife thought was "bad." He knew he had cancer, and he was satisfied with the surgery and chemotherapy he had endured. He was "cured" as far as he was concerned. Even his wife, a nurse who worked with children with cancer, agreed he was doing well, but she also "believed in science." Her research had convinced her that Don's continued health depended on changes in his lifestyle. She insisted that Don, himself, could do something to help prevent a recurrence of colon cancer.

How much was Don willing to change? Well, he came to "visit with us," to listen. He just didn't say much at first. He would respond to direct questions. Most of the time he sat with his arms crossed over his chest and stared. He was definitely a man who wanted to be somewhere else.

The night that Bob, another member of the group, began to talk about his cancer changed things for Don. Bob asked:

*If all this stuff about diet is true, why doesn't my doctor know? I'm dealing with a recurrence of bladder cancer. We've done the surgery, the radiation. I have to be checked out every few months. I asked about experimental treatment or other stuff, and the urologist said come in for regular checks, and we'd deal with whatever happens. Now you've got me thinking about things, but if I try to talk to him about relaxation and changing my diet and taking Chinese herbs, he just shrugs.*

Bob and Don were clearly experiencing the same doubts and questions. They both relied on their oncologists for expert guidance. Even the thought of questioning the doctor undermined their confidence in their treatment. Besides, they agreed, all this talk they were hearing about food and "eating with love" and nurturing yourself made them uncomfortable.

Don said he was impatient when anyone mentioned "relationships with food." He had a relationship with his wife, his dog, maybe his truck. He didn't want or need to know why he had trouble changing his diet. It was bad enough that we thought he had to eat differently, that he was even starting to think he should eat differently. Less red meat, all those fruits and vegetables, that stuff about different kinds of fats. With his job, he traveled frequently, and it was hard to control what he ate. He'd do what he had to do, but he just wanted to eat right without thinking much about it.

Of course, eating without thinking is why so many Americans are obese, and obesity, we know, is a major risk factor for cancer. Sandy said she recently realized that she became overweight eating leftovers. For years, she couldn't understand why she was so fat. So far as she could tell, she never ate more than normal; she cooked good healthy food for her family; and she indulged her love of dessert rarely. But all this thinking about food and weight and cancer made her realize she ate all the time.

She ate while shopping, she ate while cooking, and she cleaned her family's plates by consuming whatever was left. She lost no weight during or after treatment for breast cancer. However, when she joined a Center for Mind-Body Medicine "mind-body skills group" and began practicing "mindfulness" meditation—breathing slowly, paying attention to her thoughts, feelings, and sensations as they arose—a new awareness followed her into the kitchen. She told Bob and Don that you can't change your diet without being aware of what you eat, how fast you eat, and how it affects you. Her new eating habits include a low-fat, high-fiber diet and time to really enjoy her food.

## What We Know About What We Eat

Dr. Jeffrey Bland, a nutritional biochemist, has worked for 26 years in the field of clinical nutrition. Dr. Bland, a student of Dr. Linus Pauling (and, for some time, the director of Dr. Pauling's Institute), is an acknowledged leader in exploring the connections between diet and chronic illnesses and the possibilities for altering the course of disease by changing diet. He is particularly gifted at synthesizing the vast amount of available information about diet and cancer.

At CCC II, Dr. Bland gave a day-long workshop reviewing the theories and scientific evidence underlying the connection between cancer and diet. He began by pointing out that nutrition has been neglected by mainstream clinicians, in part because of an overreliance on pharmacological and technical advances in science; in part because nutrition has not been emphasized as part of medical education; and in part, as a recent article in the *Archives of Internal Medicine* pointed out, because nutrition researchers often take their data directly to an eager general public. The result is that in spite of good scientific evidence for dietary therapies and nutritional supplementation, the entire field is still regarded as somehow outside the province of most physicians.

"Let food be your medicine, and medicine your food," was one of Hippocrates' most famous dictums. It is also, we are discovering, a truth substantiated by the latest biochemical, clinical, and epidemiological findings. Nutrients, it seems, not only can directly support the body and protect us against cancer but also can mobilize our genes to better serve us. The antioxidants in foods, and in supplements, are a prime example of this first protective function of nutrition. The phytochemicals (*phyto* means "plant") in lemons, cruciferous vegetables, and soy illustrate the way food can affect genetic expression.

As the name suggests, antioxidants are substances that protect the body against oxidation, a potentially destructive process initiated by free radicals. Free radicals are molecules that are missing electrons and that actively scavenge them from other molecules, and, in the process, damage those molecules. Free radical damage affects cellular membranes and proteins as well as DNA and appears to be a factor in carcinogenesis. The antioxidants are capable of donating electrons to the free radicals. These antioxidants include vitamins A, C, E, and beta carotene; selenium; bioflavinoids, polyphenols, and resveratrol; and foods rich in them, like leafy green vegetables, carrots, citrus fruits, grapes, and green and black tea.

The effects of food on genetic expression are, Dr. Bland explained, even more remarkable and almost as pervasive. There are some genetic factors that are constitutional and cannot, so far as we know, be modified by food. The activity of a significant number of genes, however, can be modified. Food does not change the structure or genotype of these genes. It can, however, change their phenotype, the way in which these genes express themselves. And with these changes come more efficient repair of damaged chromosomes and cells and more protection against cancer-causing chemicals.

Dr. Bland explained that oranges contain over 170 different phytochemicals, a number of which can modify gene expression. One of them, "limonene," which is also present in grapefruit, stimulates the gene expression for a detoxifying enzyme called glutathione S-transferase. This enzyme protects us against certain cancer-causing chemicals by breaking them down into nontoxic derivatives.

Soy, which we discuss in more detail in Chapter 9, has similar gene-modifying properties. In some men the prostate gland produces very high levels of 5-dihydrotestosterone (DHT), a toxic derivative of testosterone that may contribute to cancer. Soy products can reduce the overstimulation of the gene that produces the enzyme that converts testosterone into this toxic derivative.

A third example of modification of genetic expression is offered by the cruciferous vegetables, including cauliflower, broccoli, cabbage, and brussels sprouts. These vegetables contain phytochemicals that, when broken down in the gut, activate genes that release a number of enzymes—including the glutathione S-transferase also stimulated by limonene—which, in turn, break down and detoxify a wide range of cancer-producing chemicals.

## Macronutrients—Fats, Carbohydrates, Protein, and Fiber

Macronutrients are compounds that are taken in large amounts and must be broken down or metabolized by the body to obtain energy or basic building material for cellular functioning. Macronutrients include fat, protein, and carbohydrates. Of these, fats—and, in particular, animal fats—have been most clearly implicated in cancer.

Dietary intake of fats—in particular, the saturated fats found in red meat and dairy products and Omega-6 polyunsaturated fats found in corn and safflower oil—has been shown, in numerous studies, to increase the incidence of gastrointestinal, prostate, breast, and colorectal cancer. We now know some of the mechanisms by which some dietary fat intake seems to promote the development and growth of cancer. These include the following:

1. High fat intake leads to increased fat tissue, and high body weight correlates to increased incidence of cancer and decreased survival in cancer patients.
2. High-fat diets decrease immune function. Reducing fat intake to 30 percent of total calories increases NK (natural killer cell) activity in the body. NK cells, tumor necrosis factor (TNF), and macrophage activity all show marked increases when dietary fats are lowered.
3. Animal fats increase the amount of prostaglandins (PGE) that are produced in many types of tumors. These messenger molecules trigger cell proliferation and depress immune competence.
4. Free radical production increases as the body metabolizes saturated fats, and this increases the possibility of damage to the DNA and subsequent malignant transformation of the cell.
5. Fats increase the bioavailability of sex hormones, which act as promoters of growth in some tumors.

Don and Bob regarded this information as an indictment of their favorite meal, more than a pound of rare beef:

*Every time we eat beef, or have a milkshake, any cancer cells become energized and aggressive? The fat molecules just run around and pass the message, "Hey, cancer cells, grow and spread!," and depress the defenses of the immune system? So these fats increase the bad guys and disarm the good guys? But don't we need some fat to live?*

Don and Bob have a handle on the problem with fat. And they are aware, as well, that we need fats to live. In fact, they were somewhat cheered when we explained that there are some fats that seem to be both generally healthful and even protective against cancer. Monounsaturated fats—found in olive oil—have been reported to decrease incidence of breast cancer (as well as protecting against heart disease), and Omega-3 fatty acids—which are found in fish—may have a similar effect, perhaps by decreasing antigenic factors and inhibiting clotting. Finally, flaxseeds not only contain large amounts of Omega-3 fatty acids, but also lignins, alcohols that have documented antitumor activity. In sum, the excessive intake of total fats can increase the risk of cancer and speed the growth and proliferation of cancer cells, but intake of Omega-3 and monounsaturated fats can help to protect us against cancer. There is an enormous amount of good evidence for reducing fats to 20–25 percent or less of our total caloric intake and for limiting or eliminating animal fats in particular.

In real life, Bob and Don need to reduce that meat portion to three or four ounces, the size of a pack of cards. They should read the labels on processed foods and vegetable oils, many of which also contain harmful unsaturated or hydrogenated fats, and use olive oil. They can eat fish, especially cold water fish like salmon and monkfish, which are a good source of Omega-3 fatty acids. And they might consider adding two tablespoons of ground flaxseed as a daily supplement.

Protein, the second of the macronutrients, is essential for growth and development; for the upkeep of DNA (which is composed of four of the amino acids that constitute protein); and for the manufacture of hormones, antibodies, and enzymes. Some amino acids are "essential," meaning that, because the body cannot synthesize them, they have to come from the diet. Dietary proteins can be "complete," which means they contain all the essential amino acids, or "incomplete." Meat, fish, cheese, eggs, and milk are complete. Grains, legumes, and leafy green vegetables are incomplete proteins.

This information is crucial for cancer patients who want to decrease intake of meat and milk products but who want to ensure that they are eating adequate amounts of protein. To get complete proteins from a largely vegetarian diet, it is necessary to combine incomplete proteins—beans with brown rice or corn, or brown rice with grains or seeds. Although there are few dietary regimens that restrict protein, we generally recommend that 15–25 percent of the diet be composed of protein, the vast majority from fish and vegetable sources.

The largest source of calories in the diet should come from carbohydrates, as much as 50–60 percent, according to Dr. Bland. The vast majority of this intake should consist of "complex" carbohydrates. Complex carbohydrates are made up of many molecules of sugars strung together. They include fiber and starches; take considerable time to digest; and provoke a slow, sustained release of insulin. Vegetables, whole grains, and beans are all complex carbohydrates. Increasing carbohydrates by eating large quantities of dark green and other brightly colored vegetables and legumes will satisfy hunger, provide phytonutrients, and contribute healthy fiber to the diet.

Simple carbohydrates include fructose (fruit sugar), sucrose (table sugar), and lactose (milk sugar). These are short-chain molecules, easily and quickly broken down and highly and quickly stimulating insulin production. Dietary sugar has been shown, in animal models, to increase the rate of tumor development and lower survival rates. Tumor cells metabolize sugar at a rate significantly greater than normal cells and, in addition, secrete factors to prevent glucose uptake by normal cells. This provokes the secretion of additional insulin, which in turn stimulates tumor growth and proliferation.

Many cancer patients report a craving for sweets, and, unfortunately, are sometimes told by uninformed physicians to eat as much as they want. In fact, we suggest limiting the amount of simple carbohydrates, and, instead, concentrating on carbohydrate intake from fresh fruits, which are also rich in vitamins, minerals, fiber, and phytonutrients. Among the fruits, we would suggest grapes, blueberries, strawberries, and cranberries, all of which contain antioxidants and ellagic acid, which stimulates the natural, programmed cell death that is called apoptosis.

Increasing intake of fruit and complex carbohydrates will also provide significant amounts of fiber. We know fiber has many functions. It reduces the risk of colorectal cancer by reducing the time the stool remains in the bowel, decreasing the concentration of carcinogens in the bowel, and supporting the growth of healthy intestinal bacteria. Dietary fiber also promotes the excretion of hormones, including estrogen and steroids. By shortening the amount of time these cancer-promoting messengers spend in the body, fiber lowers cancer risk and decreases the stimulation of hormone-sensitive tumors.

Every time we mention vegetables, fruits, and fish as an important part of cancer care, we get mixed reactions. To some people, who have already suffered so much from cancer, abandoning favorite foods seems like just another loss. Others, including Don and Bob, say these vegetarian diets seem "unnatural." One woman, an immigrant from Denmark, said she wouldn't miss meat, but restricting high-fat dairy products was against nature. *No cheese? No butter? What gives anything flavor?*

Another woman, who grew up on a cattle ranch in Texas, argued that she had read that human beings evolved as smart and adaptable because of our ability to eat anything—but especially meat. She cited, as an authority, an article in the *New England Journal of Medicine* on the "Paleolithic diet": meat, tubers, and seeds. She has a point. Meat uncontaminated by cancer promoters (such as the hormones fed to cattle) and excess fat—venison for example—is a lean and efficient source of protein. Historically, the consumption of wild meat also required substantial physical activity. No one on a Paleolithic diet became obese.

On the other hand, many of those with whom we spoke were already following some of the guidelines we were discussing and felt they did better on a vegetarian and fish diet. They liked the changes. One woman reported that eating a high-fiber, low-fat diet made her feel both lighter and stronger. Another who was battling a lifelong weight problem reported that she was losing weight without trying. Just eliminating red meat, sugar, and all processed foods, and adding more vegetables and fruits seemed to change her body's metabolism and, after a while, stopped her cravings for pastry and candy. Bob said it was all beginning to sound like a meeting for Overeaters Anonymous.

Cancer had already had an enormous impact on their lives, and now it had invaded mealtime. Yet a few examples of the elegant ways that nutrients could help them resist a recurrence of cancer and a few weeks of eating in a more healthy way seemed to make a difference. As Bob said, the choice to eat meat is always possible and, maybe, if he limits his portions and eats more fiber and fresh vegetables and fish and takes appropriate supplements, he can eat a little steak. The trick is balance and sending the right messages to the cells, he believed. He became our most avid researcher, bringing in piles of studies in his search for ways to enjoy his steak while starving any stray cancer cells.

## Micronutrients: Supplements

The use of micronutrient dietary supplements—vitamins and minerals—always causes controversy. Although antioxidants are mentioned as active, important micronutrients, present in certain foods, guidelines from the National Cancer Institute and the American Cancer Society still emphasize macronutrients and hesitate to endorse the regular use of supplements as a therapeutic intervention.

On the other hand, new data are changing attitudes and practices. For years, almost all physicians insisted that a "normal and healthy" American diet provided all the nutrition people needed, including fats, carbohydrates, proteins, and the micronutrients. This position has been gradually modified as individual variations in requirements and assimilation have been discovered. Some special groups—pregnant women, growing children, people recovering from surgery, people with cardiovascular disease, the elderly—are now encouraged to take regular, specific supplements. And, with or without medical encouragement, as many as 60 percent of all cancer patients are taking some supplement.

At CCC II we asked Dr. Bland and Dr. Daniel Nixon, a former ACS vice president and current president of the American Health Foundation, to help us sort through some of the confusion in the important and hugely controversial area of supplementation. Dr. Bland and Dr. Nixon both began by emphasizing the importance of staying within safe dosage limits. Just because some of a supplement may be beneficial—the use of the B vitamin, folic acid, for example, to promote the "methylation" of DNA and decrease the expression of tumor-promoting genes—doesn't mean "more is better." Similarly, they both emphasized the importance of "biochemical individuality": A dose of a supplement that may be adequate for most people may be inadequate for some and toxic for still others.

Drs. Bland and Nixon pointed out as well that there may be circumstances in which nutritional supplementation does conflict with other treatments. This is particularly important in the case of taking antioxidants while you are undergoing radiation or chemotherapy. Although a number of studies show that antioxidants, including vitamins A, C, and E, can enhance the effect of these treatments and decrease their side effects, some oncologists believe they may at times interfere with the therapeutic efficacy of these conventional treatments.

Finally, it's important to discuss the antioxidant vitamin A, and beta carotene, which is converted to vitamin A, which are, we believe, especially complicated cases. Many studies have shown that high levels of A and beta carotene are correlated with low incidences of a variety of cancers, including lung cancer. However, two well-known studies, the Finnish ATBC trial and the NCI CARET study, showed that supplementation with beta carotene and vitamin A actually *increased* the incidence of lung cancer among smokers and people exposed to asbestos.

There is as yet no definitive resolution to this disturbing contradiction, although some investigators believe that smokers in particular metabolize these vitamins in ways that promote cancer and that the *synthetic* beta carotene used in these studies may have actually lowered the level of other cancer-preventing carotenes. While the controversy continues, we suggest, particularly if you are a smoker, that you get your vitamin A and beta carotene from large amounts of brightly colored vegetables and fruit, and that if you do decide to take a carotene supplement it be a combination of carotenoids derived from natural sources.

With these caveats in mind, we provide below a list of suggested supplements, developed from presentations at the CCC, as *guidelines,* not as absolute authority. In fact, before we present them, we want to remind ourselves, and you, of three more things: Discuss any supplements you take with your physician; take supplements that are natural rather than synthetic; and, if at all possible, consult a nutritionist or a nutritionally oriented physician to help you develop a complete, individually tailored nutrition treatment plan.

One more point: Supplements can also be expensive, and insurance rarely covers even doctor-prescribed supplements. This is a huge problem for many of us who may be financially stretched by chronic illness and is another reason advocates of comprehensive care must also push for changes in the health delivery system. No one should do without good, proven therapies because of money.

Here, then, is our list of daily supplements:

1. A B-complex vitamin (to boost cell integrity and repair DNA damage and ensure maximal detoxification), including:
    * folate (600 mcg), B-6 (5 mg),
    * B-12 (100 mcg), and

- betaine (100–500 mg).

2. Antioxidants (to control oxidation, protect cellular
   integrity and DNA, and enhance detoxification):
   - vitamin E (400–800 IU),
   - vitamin C (500–1,000 mg),
   - beta carotene (15–30 mg),
   - manganese (5 mg),
   - zinc, to work with antioxidants and enhance
     immunity (50 mg),
   - selenium (200 mcg), and
   - and coenzyme Q10 (20–50 mg).

3. Minerals
   - calcium (which may help protect against colon
     cancer as well as bone loss), (1000–2000 mg),
   - chromium (200 mcg), and
   - magnesium (400–600 mg).

(These latter two are for glucose management, which may help
control cancer cell growth.)

There are other supplements, plant and herb extracts, that have
specific actions. Some of these natural substances that have good
supportive data for inclusion in a therapeutic diet, like soy, garlic,
and ginger, are discussed in the section on phytonutrients and in
other parts of this book.

Bob has posted this list and the various "*do's* and *don'ts* of diet"
on his refrigerator and on his computer at the office. He likes the
idea of having a plan. His goal remains to keep it simple and to
learn to balance the occasional vice (a steak) with conscientious
virtue (copious consumption of vegetables, soy prepared in strange
and hopefully tasty ways, regular antioxidant supplements). Most
of all, he wants to continue to enjoy his food. We have noticed that
the more he reads, the less he complains about changing his diet. He
is teachable, as he said.

Other patients also stressed the importance of balancing the overwhelming feelings of loss with a sense of gaining something new and

good. They have found it useful to think of adding to their diet—adding new foods, new spices, and more fruits and vegetables—rather than restricting themselves. They like experimenting with new foods and feeling encouraged and strengthened by eating what's good for them. And again and again they return to Sandy's story about learning to eat mindfully, enjoying this continually renewable, continually health-giving pleasure.

There was a moment one night, when Sandy was talking about her garden, and her first ripe tomatoes of the year:

*Sun-ripened tomatoes, smooth as satin and vibrant red in color, fit perfectly in the hand and smell like summer. Cut a slice of whole wheat bread, fresh and crusty, with the smell of yeast and warmth. Put the two together, add a little salt, and the first bite could make you swoon: High fiber, complex carbohydrates, a lycopene antioxidant—and utter joy.*

# 6

# Traditional Chinese Medicine

IN 1971 *NEW YORK TIMES* columnist James Reston described how acupuncture had relieved his pain after an emergency appendectomy. At about the same time we first began to read in the English-language edition of the *Peking Review* more detailed accounts of Chinese medicine. There were reports of successful acupuncture treatment of "deaf-mutes" and of people with arthritis and asthma, and pictures of Chinese surgical patients, slim needles in their limbs, sipping tea while surgeons probed their open chests. We also read about cancer patients who experienced pain relief, enhanced immune functioning, the disappearance of tumors and, even—although it was impossible to decipher the meaning of the word—"cures" of cancer.

Both of us felt the ground shifting slightly under our feet as we raced through digests of these studies. What we were reading seemed so improbable from the point of view of Western medicine: Children deaf from birth or early childhood were hearing again, people crippled with arthritis who could walk, asthmatics who were abandoning medication on which they had long depended, and people with metastatic cancer "cured."

The methodological flaws in the studies gave us pause. Most were not controlled, and words like "cure" were never defined. The possibility that all this was the result of a placebo response—the power of belief in people convinced of the correctness of the ancient treatment—was never far from our skeptical minds. On the other hand, we could understand that the Chinese, with a billion souls to succor, didn't have the economic luxury to use more careful methodologies, and that the translations might be flawed.

Still, unless we labeled the whole enterprise as fraudulent, we had to be impressed with the numbers—often thousands of patients in a single study—and the results. The placebo problem continued to concern us, until we read veterinary studies, and in particular one on the successful acupuncture treatment of "laminitis," inflammation of the hooves, in oxen. Oxen, we knew, were unlikely to be much influenced by the acupuncturist's belief—or their own—in the power of his needles. Even allowing for poor study design and some exaggeration, something positive and promising, and quite mysterious, was clearly going on.

Nothing in our medical backgrounds had prepared us for this technique or these findings. How could needles in the body relieve pain or improve circulation or stop intractable hiccups or abort an asthma attack? Then we began to experience acupuncture ourselves. It relaxed and energized us, relieved long-standing muscle and joint pain, improved circulation, even helped a crippled dog named Zeke to walk again.

We had to find out what was going on, and began a 30-year study—first of acupuncture; then of the Chinese moving meditations, *tai chi* and *qi gong*; and then of Chinese herbs and nutritional therapies, and of *tui na,* the Chinese version of massage and osteopathic manipulation. More recently we—and many of our colleagues—have turned our attention to the power of Chinese medicine to make a very real difference for people with cancer, and to the possibility of making the approach and methods of this 2,500-year-old healing system an integral part of modern America's comprehensive cancer care.

## Traditional Chinese Medicine

The world of traditional Chinese medicine (TCM) is indissolubly connected to the larger world we live in. The principles according to which our bodies and minds move and maintain their balance are the same as those that govern the form and function of the natural world. Changes in us reflect and depend on the changes in that world. We live, when we are healthy, in and according to the *tao*, "the way." It is like a river, flowing, ever changing, ever new. And it is, as Lao-tzu, its great sage and poet, wrote, also impossible to define: "The way that can be described is not the way." Definition, or even its attempt, removes us from the flow. Experience, made possible by our hands and eyes and hearts, opens us to it.

The tao expresses itself in the world in polarities that are complementary. The Chinese call them *yin* and *yang*. Yin means "the shady side of the hill." It is feminine, damp, dark, slow, and deep, and closer to the bottom or tail of an organism than to the top, or head. Yang, the "sunny side of the hill," is masculine, dry, bright, quick, and superficial, and closer to the top than the bottom. Everything on our planet, our entire universe, including the organs in our body, the pathogens that afflict us, the moods we experience, and the remedies we use to treat cancer, may be described as either yin or yang.

The yang organs are hollow, like the stomach; the yin organs solid, like the spleen. Yang diseases are usually acute and are characterized by fever, sweating, constipation, a dry mouth, dark urine, heavy breathing, a rapid pulse, and irritability. People suffering from yin conditions feel chilly and have loose bowels, shallow breathing, a slow pulse, and a feeling of lethargy. These conditions are usually chronic. Cancer may be predominantly yang in early stages, when tumors, bleeding, and fever first appear and yin in later stages, with weakness, fluid accumulation, and fatigue.

Yin and yang are not, however, static. Yin becomes yang, as the night gives way to the day, and yang in turn becomes yin, as the light yields to the dark. Each contains the other within it, just as each half of the famous black and white yin-yang symbol contains a small circle of the other's color: The first glimmerings of dawn are there in the darkest night and the acute injury gives way to the chronic nagging pain. Each of the polarities is defined in relation to the other: The chest is high or yang in relation to the abdomen, yin to the head's yang.

Human beings are a field in which the eternal play of yin and yang takes place. We are also, simultaneously, and in the kind of paradox that is so prevalent in the Chinese worldview, mediators between the heavenly destiny that is yang and the earthly nature that is yin.

The Chinese way of knowing is not primarily analytical. The verb *to know* is constructed of characters that represent both "the tao" and "to know." To know is to know the tao, and knowing comes through living in and through the tao. The first Chinese physicians were monks. They lived in a pastoral world, alert to the ebb and flow of nature. They practiced meditation, going within to experience the energy, the *qi*, that animated all the processes in their minds and bodies. They came, so far as we are able to tell, to know the bodies they lived in not primarily by dissection of the dead or experimentation on the living but through meditation, introspection, and observation. They came to sense the subtle connections between the organs in their bodies and the times of day, the seasons of the year, the colors of the spectrum, and the plants and animals among which they lived.

The Chinese medicine we are now learning about and practicing in the West comes from the experience, several thousand years ago, of these adepts, and from the refinements made by all the generations of their students since then. It is based on a system of substances, influences, and categories that is not easily accessible to contemporary westerners but that would have been quite comprehensible to Hippocratic or Galenic physicians, who used the words "humors" and "airs," "pneuma" or spirit, and "psyche" or soul.

There are, the Chinese tell us, three treasures: *shen* (mind or spirit), *qi* (energy), and *jing* (essence). Although these three are the fundamental substances of life, qi is regarded as the most basic, the one of which the others are manifestations. The written character for qi suggests its dynamic capacity for change; it includes the characters for "uncooked rice" and for "steam"—for a solid substance, the vapor that its cooking produces, and the process of transformation that produces the vapor.

Qi is "the root of a human being." It is the refined energy that nourishes the body and mind, as well as the dynamic functioning of all the organs. It circulates constantly, through the lines on the body, the "meridians" on which the acupuncture points lie, energizing the organs in turn. It is also the nutrition that is extracted from food, the process of nourishing the internal organs, and the force that propels the blood and animates the lungs. Qi is the shield that protects the person against adverse climates, microorganisms, the immune insults, genetic damage, and stress that may be related to the development of cancer.

*Jing* is the essence. In its "pre-heaven" manifestation it is the precious substance that nourishes the embryo during pregnancy and helps sustain the organism throughout life. In its "post-heaven" form it is extracted from food and stored largely in the kidneys, where it is said to sustain growth, development, regeneration, and reproduction. It nourishes the mind and protects the body. Jing and qi are the foundation of the more subtle and refined *shen*, or spirit. Shen, which resides in the heart, depends on them and will flourish if they are healthy and abundant; it will decline if they are not.

In addition to these three, the Chinese describe two other vital substances, blood and moisture, or bodily fluids. Blood, regarded as a dense form of qi, flows with it throughout the body, nourishing organs. Both blood and bodily fluids are extracted from food. The fluids are repeatedly purified and transformed into urine, sweat, saliva, and all of the body's other lubricants and secretions, and these in turn lend the tissues their suppleness. TCM has a thoroughly integrated vision of mind, body, and spirit: "Where shen leads," it proclaims, "qi follows, and where qi goes, blood flows."

The "eight principles" of TCM are ways to organize and distinguish among the patterns in human functioning and to describe different kinds of disharmony. Yin and yang are both the most fundamental of these principles and descriptions of the first of four paired polarities. Others are "excess" and "deficiency," "interior" and "exterior," and "hot" and "cold." Thus, there can be a "lung yin deficiency" or "stomach heat and qi deficiency." There are internal causes of disease in the emotions, as in sadness affecting the lungs and depleting their qi. External causes are climatic, as in dampness producing lethargy and edema.

The body's organs—the heart, lungs, liver, kidneys, and so on—are the sources of the vital substances—blood and fluid—and the locations in which imbalances may be found. The Chinese regard these organs as like and yet different from the organs we see when we open our anatomy books. They partake of something larger, a fundamental category of experience variously called a "phase" or "element," in which they are linked to specific emotions, times of day, seasons, colors, tastes, and sounds. There are five of these elements: wood, fire, earth, metal, and water. Each element is connected to and emblematic of an organ, for example, the liver of wood and the heart of fire. Each element nourishes the one that succeeds it—as wood feeds fire or as the mother feeds the child—and each governs or controls another element. Fire, for example, controls metal.

Each element has its own particular picture. Metal, for example, is the element of fall. Its emotions are apprehension and sorrow; its qi is highest between the hours of 3:00 and 7:00 in the morning, when the associated organs, the lungs and colon, are said to be functioning at their maximum strength. Metal "types"—similar in some ways to those Western psychologists describe as "repressive copers"—tend to restrict their emotions and suffer when events elude their control. Metal is the mother of water (water condenses on metal), and it controls (cuts) wood. Asthma is often (though not always) a "metal" condition, as are irritable bowel syndrome, colitis, and anxiety. The imbalances in the metal organs (constipation or poor breathing patterns) may contribute to acne or eczema.

The Chinese physician assesses the state of the fundamental substances, the eight principle characteristics, and the vitality of the organs by carefully listening to, observing, and touching his patient. The voice tells one story—the metal type, or the person with a metal ailment, speaks with a crying sound. The shape and color of the various parts of the face and the smell of the body give other information.

According to the Chinese, each part of the body is a microcosm of the whole, a map on which the signs of imbalance may be read. To the Chinese the tongue, barely noticed now in the West, offers a window on the body's recent functioning and long-standing problems. It size, shape, fissures, furrows, coats, textures, and colors and its degree of moistness and dryness yield data about which substance and organ may be malfunctioning. The lungs, which sit in the chest, are read toward the front of the tongue, while the functioning of the colon and kidneys, which are lower in the body, can be determined by the appearance of the root of the tongue. A bright red tongue signals excess heat, a pale one may indicate deficient blood, deficient heat, or excess cold.

Areas of tenderness and tightness in the belly, sounds, discolorations, and hollows there will yield other clues about blockages in the flow of qi, blood, and moisture. The pulses, the most subtle and complex of the diagnostic guides, will fill in the gaps, telling the skilled practitioner—by their size and contours, their solidity, tension, or hollowness—not only which organ and substance is disordered but what illnesses have afflicted and may afflict the patient.

## TCM and Cancer

As early as the eleventh century B.C. there were drawings of tumors on "oracle bones" and turtle shells in China. By 200 B.C. the Chinese texts were emphasizing the hardness of tumors and their common origin in the impaired circulation of qi and blood. The texts describe congestion as the first stage in this process, stagnation the second, and accumulation the third. According to the ancient physicians, both external and internal factors could set this process in motion, including intense cold and deep and prolonged sadness. Ultimately, this process of accumulation distorts the circulation of qi, disengages the smooth functioning of yin and yang, and leads to a lack of harmony and control in the entire body.

The traditional Chinese medicinal treatment of cancer is based on the principle of *fu zheng gu ben*. Roughly speaking, fu zheng means strengthening what is correct, the qi, the forces in the body regulating normal healthy development. Gu ben refers to strengthening and enhancing the processes of regeneration and repair, which Chinese medicine locates in the kidney. Traditional treatment includes removing toxins that may contribute to cancer, increasing the flow of blood and qi, removing undesirable accumulations of tissue that are the tumor, and restoring self-regulation and balance among jing, shen, and qi. The means that are used—acupuncture, herbal and nutritional therapies, *tai chi, qi gong, tui na,* and counseling—are each designed to further one or more aspects of this process.

Although there are general principles of treatment, TCM individualizes the therapeutic approach to each cancer patient. Even when the organ of origin, the pathological diagnosis, and the stage are exactly the same in Western terms, the TCM clinical picture may be quite different. For example, one patient's cervical cancer may be characterized primarily by "qi stagnation," while another might manifest "liver and yin deficiency." Each picture represents a different physiological and psychological state. Each demands the use of different acupuncture points, a different combination of herbs, different sets of *qi gong* exercises, and an altogether different style of counseling. And each is expected to—and, as it turns out, does—have a significantly different prognosis.

## The Marriage of Chinese and Western Medicine

Since the 1970s, the revival of interest in TCM in China has been accompanied and stimulated by modern Western research. Chinese physicians and researchers who are well trained in TCM and Western medicine have begun to use sophisticated modern methodologies—in vitro and in vivo studies, epidemiological surveys, prospective and randomized controlled trials—to study both the effectiveness and the means of action of traditional treatments. At the same time, approximately 20,000 North Americans, many trained as physicians, have learned about and begun to practice acupuncture and Chinese medicine. Some are now undertaking studies on their own—and at medical schools—on the effectiveness of TCM.

In cancer care there has been a significant focus on the benefits of integrating TCM with conventional Western treatments: acupuncture, herbs, *and* chemotherapy. In the following discussion we sum-

marize some of the most promising developments and then give recommendations for the way in which this medical system, and its
practitioners and techniques, can be successfully integrated into
your program of comprehensive cancer care.

## Acupuncture

For most westerners acupuncture is the door to Chinese medicine.
Its results can be swift, dramatic, and palpable: an immediate decrease in pain, a feeling of relaxation, a diminution in craving for
narcotics. It is relatively easy for Western health professionals to
learn the basics of symptomatic treatment (although a very long
study indeed to become a master), and there is significant research
to validate both acupuncture's mode of action and its efficacy.

At Comprehensive Cancer Care II, Dr. Ming Tian, the physician-
acupuncturist who treats patients at NIH's Clinical Center, high-
lighted some of the ways in which acupuncture can contribute to
cancer care. He reminded us that research done in the West as well
as in China has shown that acupuncture, properly used, releases
pain-reducing endorphins; that it exerts a significant effect on the
metabolism of serotonin, a neurotransmitter that powerfully affects
both pain perception and mood; and that it can enhance circulation
and immune functioning.

The most extensive and careful studies on the clinical uses of
acupuncture, however, have been conducted on its capacity to treat
the nausea and vomiting produced by chemotherapy. These studies
are consistent and impressive enough so that the NIH itself, at a recent "Consensus Conference," recommended the use of this approach. It is interesting to note that most of these studies on treating
nausea and vomiting were done using a single acupuncture point,
"Pericardium 6," on the volar, or palm, side of the forearm, about
three fingerbreadths up from the crease at the wrist. This point,
which has also been used to treat seasickness and the nausea of first-
trimester pregnancy, is highly potent and easy to use.

From the perspective of randomized controlled studies (P-6 can be
compared with a single "sham," or ineffective, point at another

location), this is a good method. But, as useful as P-6 is, it is likely that we would get still better results if we used multiple points tailored to each person's clinical picture. There are, in Chinese medicine, at least 10 distinct clinical pictures of nausea and vomiting induced by chemotherapy. Each has its own set of required points. In practice, if you were to see a skilled acupuncturist, he or she would choose the points that precisely match *your* clinical picture.

Although studies on acupuncture use in other aspects of cancer treatment are not as definitive as those on nausea and vomiting, acupuncture is an important and recognized part of clinical practice with cancer patients. According to Dr. Ming and many other practitioners, as well as our own experience, acupuncture can reliably

- Decrease pain and induce relaxation, even when other approaches don't work.
- Improve mood and energy levels.
- Treat the intractable hiccups that sometimes occur in cancer patients.

### Brad's "Cool Treatment"

Fifteen-year-old Brad's experience is illustrative—and increasingly common.

Brad was being treated at a comprehensive cancer center for his high-grade astrocytoma, a very threatening tumor originating in brain cells. His pediatrician, neurologist, and neurosurgeon had all the right credentials, all the certifications and training and experience to treat Brad's brain cancer. He was responding well to aggressive treatment: surgery, radiation, and chemotherapy. The doctors were hopeful and reassuring. Surgery had removed most of the tumor, and the latest brain scan showed no new growth. The cancer was not yet fully defeated—it could recur—but the doctors felt Brad was doing well.

The problem was that Brad felt horrible. What he saw in the mirror every day was a very sick person: ashen, thin, trembling, and frightened. He had no appetite, no energy, no hair, and problems with balance and coordination. He wasn't eating, he had trouble sleeping, he wasn't able to read or concentrate on anything. Going to school, hanging with his friends, music, computer games—all seemed impossible tasks. Brad constantly worried about his potency and whether he would grow taller and if he would ever get body hair, but kept these concerns to himself. The cancer might have been defeated, but Brad believed the cancer and the lifesaving but toxic treatment had left him wounded, perhaps beyond repair, and exhausted. He had no sense of victory, just a feeling of bone tiredness and despair.

Brad was genuinely polite, self-effacing, and stoic. He deeply appreciated his parents' efforts and didn't want to worry them further. But he was becoming desperate, too desperate to worry about hurting their feelings by challenging his therapeutic regimen. He knew he sounded ungrateful for his survival, asking for more from everyone, but he was scared. He had seen a TV show about acupuncture, learned that it could help nausea and vomiting and pain, and had heard something about old people getting more energy from acupuncture. Well, acupuncture looked weird, but the people on the show seemed happy with it, and he felt like he was a hundred.

Linda and Dave had been so pleased with Brad's remission that they had tended to ignore the side effects of his treatment. Now, they were shocked and dismayed by their son's desperation: Was Brad's life forever diminished by the interventions that made his life possible? Somehow they felt they had forgotten to pay attention to all of Brad—his body, mind, and spirit—while the cancer in his brain was being treated. Chinese medicine sounded strange to them, too, but they would do anything they could to help their son.

A friend recommended a medical doctor who used TCM in his practice. Brad was enthusiastic, and his parents felt that having a "regular" doctor who had also studied Chinese medicine would make the experience less threatening. They called and made an appointment.

The doctor's office and his diplomas were immediately reassuring to Linda and Dave. Brad was more interested in the acupuncture charts, full of mysterious Chinese characters and lines tracing the flow of energy in the body. He found it "cool."

Brad insisted he wanted to see this doctor alone. He wanted this experience for himself. He had spent one and one-half years never being alone. He was 15 years old. It was time, he decided, to take some responsibility for himself. After all, he was the one who asked for acupuncture.

Brad began receiving regular acupuncture treatments, started a regimen of herbal remedies that made him groan—more medicine!—and promised to improve his diet. Later, the TCM doctor suggested Brad start *tai chi* to improve his stamina and balance. Brad began to put on weight. School became less exhausting and there was time and energy to hang with his friends. Six months later, he feels hopeful, stronger, more at home in a body that seems to be growing a little more graceful—and he is starting to think about college and the future.

Brad still isn't himself, he says, but he thinks his experience with the cancer and the TCM is helping him to be stronger, maybe even a more interesting person. There's this girl in his history class . . . she had a headache and he showed her the acupressure point to make it go away, and she wants to go to *tai chi* class, too.

### Herbal Remedies

Chinese herbal medicine is a vast field, and a fertile one for cancer treatment. There are more than 7,000 plants (and animal parts and minerals) that are used therapeutically in China. Because these substances are customarily used in combination, there is an almost infinite variety of medicinal preparations.

The herbs—and the combinations—that are used in cancer treatment have a number of significant direct modes of action, including immune stimulation, anti-tumor activity, inhibition of chemotherapy-induced immunosuppression, enhancement of circulation, and inhibition of platelet aggregation and clotting. Other actions include stress reduction, mood and energy enhancement, and reduction of the nausea and vomiting of chemotherapy.

Some herbs have one major effect: *Salvia*, for example, is particularly useful in increasing circulation, while ginger reduces nausea and vomiting. Other herbs have a variety of effects. *Glycyrrhizae* (licorice) has anti-inflammatory and anti-tumor properties and increases natural killer cell activity. *Atractylodes* has anti-tumor and clot-reducing activity, improves learning and memory, reduces stress, modulates cellular metabolic processes, and enhances white blood cell formation.

*Panax ginseng*, which is used in many cancer-treating formulas, is known as an "adaptogen." In addition to its primary effects on cancer—inhibiting tumor growth, enhancing immunity, and inhibiting platelet aggregation and the immune suppression of chemotherapy—it helps the body to deal more effectively with environmental and psychological stressors, increases overall strength and endurance, and restores balance.

Because only abstracts, and not complete translations, of most of the Chinese studies are available, it is hard to evaluate them with full confidence. Nevertheless, the results appear promising and, indeed, exciting. A few of the Chinese studies have compared herbal treatment with chemotherapy or radiation. Most, however, have focused on comparisons of people treated conventionally with, or without, additional herbal therapy.

In one study, a group of 188 patients with advanced nasopharyngeal cancer (a quite common type in China) were assigned randomly to groups that received either radiation or radiation together with "destagnating" (circulation enhancing) herbs. The 5-year survival rate of the destagnation group was 53 percent, compared to 37 percent of the control group. In another study, a traditional herbal combination of ginseng, *Atractylodes*, *Poria*, and *Glycyrrhizae* was used, with and without chemotherapy, for patients with primary liver cancer. The 5-year survival in the treatment group increased from 6 to 23 percent.

A study of 285 people with a variety of kinds of cancer that had metastasized to the lymph nodes above the collar bones showed similar results. The patients were divided among those who took radiation by itself, chemotherapy alone, and only Chinese medicine;

those who took radiation therapy plus Chinese medicine; and those who took chemotherapy and Chinese medicine. Neither radiation nor chemotherapy by itself produced a significant decrease (25 percent or more) in lymph node size. Traditional Chinese medicine by itself produced significant shrinkage in only 12.5 percent of the patients, whereas traditional Chinese medicine *plus* chemotherapy produced shrinkage in 55 percent, and TCM *plus* radiotherapy produced shrinkage in 75 percent.

## Comprehensive Cancer Care Studies

The studies on Chinese herbs presented at Comprehensive Cancer Care I and II were carefully done and presented, in their entirety, in English. These studies confirmed the kinds of findings that are coming out of China and offered models for careful research. We believe they will help pave the way for the inclusion of these and other Chinese herbal combinations in the comprehensive cancer care of Americans.

Dr. Sophie Chen's experience using a combination of traditional Chinese herbs and the Western herb *Serrenoa ripens* (saw palmetto) is discussed in detail in Chapter 9. Here we focus on Dr. Yan Su's work on atrophic gastritis, a precancerous condition, and on Dr. Alexander Sun's use of "nontoxic" vegetables and herbs to treat non-small cell lung carcinoma.

Yan Su is currently a researcher at Georgetown Medical School's Lombardi Cancer Center. While he was still in China, he studied the herbal treatment of atrophic gastritis, an inflammatory disorder of the stomach characterized by a decrease in the number and thickness of cells in its lining. In China people have a very high incidence of atrophic gastritis, which is a condition that is almost certainly precancerous: Approximately 10 to 15 percent of Chinese people with atrophic gastritis will develop gastric cancer, and 80 percent of those with gastric cancer have a history of atrophic gastritis.

Using a mixture of traditional Chinese herbs, Dr. Su and his colleagues were able to significantly increase the thickness of the stomach lining in rats in whom atrophic gastritis had been created. In humans—matching two different herbal mixtures to two different clinical pictures—70 percent of all atrophic gastritis patients showed a good response: Damaged cells disappeared and healthy ones regrew. At the same time, the treatment—which did not contain conventional antibiotics—was successful, in the majority of cases, in eliminating *Helicobacter pylori*, a bacterial infection that has been implicated in stomach ulcers and may also play a significant role in atrophic gastritis.

Dr. Su's study gave clear evidence of the use of herbal mixtures to help prevent one precancerous condition from becoming cancer. It also may have implications for preventing other kinds of cancer, as well as for the treatment of gastric ulcers.

Alexander Sun, a biochemist who has worked at the Rockefeller Institute and Mount Sinai Hospital as well as Yale Medical School, originally developed a mixture of therapeutic foods and herbs to treat his elderly mother. In 1984, Mrs. Sun was one of approximately 120,000 people in the United States who each year is diagnosed with non-small cell lung carcinoma. Her tumor was Stage IV and the prognosis grim.

Each day Mrs. Sun drank the remedy her son developed, which contains large amounts of soy, shiitake mushrooms, *Panax ginseng*, ginger, and a number of other ingredients. Her life expectancy with Stage IV tumor with conventional treatment would most likely have been less than a year (4–10 months is average). On her son's soup (there *is* a pun here), she has been alive, well, and apparently tumor-free for more than 15 years.

Dr. Sun was understandably impressed. His mother's improvement encouraged him to test his soup on other people with cancer. At Comprehensive Cancer Care II he presented a carefully designed and implemented new study, which has subsequently been published in the peer-reviewed journal *Nutrition and Cancer*. All patients in this study had biopsy and x-ray confirmed Stage III or Stage IV nonsmall cell lung carcinoma. All were treated with conventional therapies, including radiation, surgery, and/or chemotherapy, according to selection criteria established by their physicians. More than half of the patients agreed to ingest Dr. Sun's soup; the others, with similar stage cancers, did not.

The results were impressive. The patients who took Sun's soup along with conventional therapies had a significantly better quality of life, less drug toxicity, and far less weight loss, even when they stopped the soup (because of its taste or its tendency to cause bloating) before the entire treatment period was over. Most important of all, they lived longer, an average of 15 months, rather than 4 months in the control group. Although the numbers in the study are small, the threefold difference in time of survival and the other benefits are striking as well as statistically significant. After his presentation at Comprehensive Cancer Care II, the National Cancer Institute agreed to review Dr. Sun's data and help him implement a randomized clinical trial.

As impressive and important as Dr. Sun's work is, it only hints at the power of herbs as a complement (or, in some otherwise untreatable cases, perhaps an alternative) to conventional therapy. As Dr. Sun pointed out, he initially developed his mixture for his mother and was particularly concerned that none of the ingredients have any toxicity. It is entirely possible that using more potent traditional food and herbal combinations, or formulating combinations individually tailored to each person, will yield even better results.

## Tai Chi and Qi Gong

The *tai chi* that Brad learned is a graceful moving meditation that tens of millions of Chinese practice each morning. These exercises are believed to enhance and prolong life by facilitating and enhancing the circulation of qi. This may or may not be true. We do, however, know that *tai chi* brings suppleness to the limbs, oxygenation to the blood, and greater stability and balance to all, and particularly to the elderly.

*Qi gong* ("gong" means circulation or movement) has thousands of different forms. Each combines meditation and imagery with breathing techniques and movements. There are basically two different kinds of *qi gong*: "internal," or "soft" *qi gong,* and "external," or "hard" *qi gong*. Internal *qi gong* includes exercises that one does to enhance one's own physiological functioning and address particular illnesses, as well as exercises designed to promote harmonious coexistence with the nature within and around us.

External *qi gong* refers to the transfer of qi from one person to another, usually through hands held close to or touching the body of the person to whom qi is transferred. External *qi gong* is a type of "energy healing" similar to, but more specific and perhaps more potent than, the "therapeutic touch" that thousands of U.S. nurses practice.

Although *qi gong* has been widely practiced in one form or another for several thousand years, modern interest in its use for cancer was prompted by the experience and teachings of a Chinese woman named Guo Lin. In the 1970s Madame Lin, whose uterine cancer had been unrelieved by six operations, created the "new *qi gong*," a system of internal *qi gong* that includes a number of "walking" exercises that, she claims, cured her. Her success and her charismatic personality energized a number of other Chinese, many with advanced cancer, to try her method. The results often were, in the words of one of the Chinese medical researchers who studied them, "astonishing."

In the past 20 years both forms of *qi gong* have been practiced and studied as therapeutic modalities for cancer. Studies on external *qi gong* on human cancer cell lines, and on mice and other animals with implanted tumors, are impressive, and abstracts are available for several dozen of them. One study from the First Medical College in Guang Su showed that mice with implanted tumors that were treated by a "*qi gong* master" lived 89 percent longer than identical, untreated mice; treatment also significantly increased both the T lymphocyte counts and the level of the enzyme superoxide dismutase in the peripheral blood. Other animal studies on external *qi gong* have shown decreases in tumor size, prevention of metastases, and enhancement of immune and other defensive functions as well as destruction of cancer cells.

The studies of both external and internal *qi gong* in humans with cancer are neither as straightforward nor as impressive. There are no comparisons, for example, between other kinds of caring or touch and the use of external *qi gong* or between other kinds of exercise and internal *qi gong*. Still, the regular practice of internal *qi gong*, for 1 or 2 hours a day over a period of 3 to 6 months, seems fairly reliably to improve strength, enhance mood, increase appetite, and promote weight gain in cancer patients, as well as to enhance some measures of immune functioning.

## A Few Words of Summary

When we look over the evidence that is accumulating and our own 30 years of clinical experience, we are impressed with the utility of Chinese medicine—and still more, with its promise for both general health care and cancer treatment. At the present time the available evidence on treatment and side effects makes us comfortable in recommending that TCM be integrated into comprehensive cancer care, along with mind-body and nutritional therapies and group support, and conventional surgery, chemotherapy, and radiation.

We feel confident in suggesting that you consider

1. Acupuncture as a primary treatment for the nausea and vomiting of chemotherapy and as part of a comprehensive program to enhance well-being and levels of energy; to improve appetite and mood; and to decrease pain, anxiety, and discomfort.
2. *Qi gong* exercises—internal *qi gong*—as a pleasurable way to improve general physiological functioning and to decrease the side effects of treatment. Internal *qi gong* appears to increase energy, and, indeed, make a significant contribution to quality of life, enhancing the body's capacity to deal with cancer as well as its treatment. External *qi gong* may also be helpful.
3. Chinese herbal therapies. Optimally, you would work with a highly qualified practitioner, a physician trained in

both Chinese and Western medicine who is familiar with the conventional treatment of cancer as well as the use of herbs. Increasingly, there are also well-trained oriental medical doctors (OMDs), including many westerners, who are grounded in Western science and highly trained in Chinese medicine. These licensed practitioners can carefully individualize Chinese herbal treatments to your specific needs and work with your oncologist to successfully combine this treatment with radiation and chemotherapy as well as surgery.

For those who do not have access to a highly trained practitioner, we recommend the use of standardized and generally nontoxic combinations like Dr. Sun's soup and Dr. Chen's well-researched PC-SPES. Although Dr. Sun's major research has been on non-small cell lung carcinoma, it appears that his preparation has benefits for other tumors. Dr. Chen is currently studying variations of her formula that can meet the needs of people with a variety of kinds of cancer.

Some oncologists are already encouraging the study and use of Chinese herbs. Many, however, are still fearful of unspecified kinds of interference between the herbs and radiation and chemotherapy. Our best reading of the Chinese literature, as well as presentations at Comprehensive Cancer Care I and II, indicate that this is not a common occurrence. In fact, as we've explained, the best research has shown that using herbs *appropriately* in combination with chemotherapy and radiation significantly *enhances* the effectiveness of these therapies. We recommend that you inform your oncologist about what you are planning to do and ask him or her to speak with your TCM practitioner, or with Dr. Chen or Dr. Sun.

Finally, we suggest that you might want to explore the Chinese worldview, with its deep, reassuring understanding of the importance of balance among body, mind, and spirit, and its appreciation of our own capacity to restore and enjoy this balance. Ultimately, Chinese medicine encourages us not only to survive cancer and feel better, but also to live more in harmony with our true nature.

# 7

# Immunomodulating Substances: Coley's Toxins, Mistletoe, MTH–68/H

THE WORD *IMMUNE* comes from the Latin *immunis,* or "free from servitude." Our immune system, our body's defender, helps keep us free from the destruction of external invaders—bacteria, viruses, parasites, and foreign substances like pollen and dust—and helps destroy damaged cells that threaten us from within—the cells of cancer.

A bacterial invasion in, say, the throat, gives us an intimate experience of the immune response at full power. The invading bacteria are identified as intruders. Molecules on the surface of the cells of the bacteria, which carry its identifying code, act as "antigens," and stimulate our immune response. Proteins called antibodies are manufactured by lymphocytes and recognize, mark, and target the bacterial antigens. Macrophages and neutrophils rush to the spot to engulf, digest, and clean up the microbes and any harmful toxins they might secrete. Lymph nodes in the neck may swell with the production of immunity-inducing cells and as the lymphatic vessels drain the infected area in the throat. Other immune cells from the bone marrow (B cells) and the thymus (T cells) may be mobilized. The immune response destroys the invader and creates an immune system memory of the invader's specific antigen identifier.

Many of the symptoms we feel when the immune response is activated are signs that the body is defending itself. These symptoms can include fever, which makes the temperature of the body dangerous to bacteria; reddening; swelling (as the *white blood* cells crowd the intruders); and pain. Over time, the symptoms lessen. Our temperature returns to normal, pain and soreness disappear, and our voice is restored. The immune system has performed its function, healthy equilibrium is reestablished, and the threat of the bacterial infection is over.

The power of the immune system to protect us against exterior invaders has been well known since the English physician Edward Jenner prepared a vaccine against small pox in the late eighteenth century. In 1908 the great biologist Paul Ehrlich suggested the nature of the immune system's protective effect against cancer. Ehrlich hypothesized that cancer cells were constantly being created, and then destroyed, by an immune system that recognizes them as "different." Sixty years later Sir Macfarland Burnet named this process "immune surveillance" and declared that it operated through the agency of lymphocytes and other cells that the immune system produces.

Currently, most scientists believe, as Burnet did, that the body constantly produces cancer cells but that its protective functions usually contain and destroy them. It is, in fact, mathematically logical to assume that, with 10 trillion cells dividing and multiplying, with all the DNA replication that must occur, mistakes will happen. It also makes sense that, to survive, our systems would have many protective abilities. And, indeed, we do: defects in the DNA can be detected by a built-in mechanism of recognition and repair that is active during the process of cell division; if the damage is irreparable, certain signals are released from within the damaged cell or from surrounding cells that induce cell suicide, called apoptosis. Similarly, some cancer cells display tumor antigens, proteins that elicit a response from the white blood cells—T lymphocytes, natural killer cells, and macophages—of the immune system. These "failsafe" mechanisms are an intrinsic part of the design, much as our satellite systems are programmed to self-destruct if certain things go wrong.

All too often, however, these fail-safe mechanisms do fail. Sometimes, when people are taking immune suppressing drugs to facilitate an organ transplant or control certain degenerative diseases, the immune system is so debilitated and damaged that cancerous cells are able to proliferate. Conventional cancer treatments—chemotherapy and radiation—are likewise immune-impairing and themselves potentially carcinogenic.

At other times, people with apparently competent immune systems also develop cancer. Even though the cancer cells are different—and are potentially deadly to the organism—our body does not recognize the threat or deploy effective protective measures. The cancer cells have disguised themselves by masking their tumor-specific antigens or have disarmed the defenses massing against them.

Even before Ehrlich's time, clinicians and researchers had begun to experiment with ways to mobilize the immune system, to deal with the cancer cells—and tumors—that had escaped natural surveillance. These efforts to stimulate, strengthen, or restore immune system function—with herbs, foods, or other physical agents or other strategies—are called "immunomodulating," and the therapies themselves are called immunotherapies.

We have talked about mind-body techniques—meditation, relaxation, and guided imagery—that enhance immune system response. We have also shared data on support groups that enhance the quality of life of their members, increase their numbers of T cells and natural killer cells, and prolong their life. We—along with many of the researchers—believe, but do not know for sure, that there may be a causal connection among these findings: that these self-care strategies, and group support, may improve quality of life and thereby enhance immunity, and that better immune functioning may lead, at times, to better defenses against cancer and longer life.

In this chapter we discuss some of the biological therapies that are designed to enhance immunity, that encourage the cells and processes already at work within the body to better recognize and combat cancer. Unlike chemotherapy and radiation, which attack cancer cells but also weaken our defenses against them, these agents and substances hold out the promise of stimulating the protective mechanisms of our own immune system and of enhancing, as well, our general physiological functioning.

## Julie's Quest

Julie was in Washington, D.C., on a quest. She flew in from Iowa and ignored the monuments, museums, and the alpha citizens of the city, our nation's political leaders. All Julie wanted to know was how to save her own life.

Six months before, Julie had noticed blood in her urine and had visited her gynecologist. A healthy and busy working mother, she assumed nothing was really wrong. *Just being conscientious,* Julie said. *I'm 32 years old, I've had a few bladder infections, I thought this was the same sort of thing. Of course, nothing in my life has been the same since I noticed those few strands of red in the bathroom. Within two weeks I was lab-tested and CAT-scanned into a new world: I had renal cell cancer, a Stage III cancer that started in my kidney. Surgery was immediately scheduled, and now I have one kidney and a 5-year survival chance of 5 to 40 percent, depending on who you talk to.*

Julie came to the Comprehensive Cancer Care conference because she had learned that renal cancer is particularly responsive to therapies employing immune system responses, including interferon alpha and interleukin 2. After her kidney was removed, she was told that more conventional treatments, although available, were not likely to significantly improve her chances of survival. She was concerned that if she tried radiation and chemotherapy, which would damage her immune system, it would forever limit other possibilities. She wanted to know more, now, about immunotherapies before she made further treatment decisions.

When we met Julie at the Comprehensive Cancer Care conference, she was investigating an experimental clinical trial, sponsored by the National Institutes of Health, that was using a combination of chemotherapy and either interleukin or interferon—she wasn't sure which—and continuing her exploration of other options she'd found on the Internet. She told us her family was very supportive, and her church friends were praying, but she just knew she had to do more. She was at the CCC to learn about other immune therapies, to ask questions, and to find some hopeful messages.

Julie has a very clear idea of who she is. She is short, wears sensible shoes, and chooses clothes that emphasize her solid, blocky body. She wears her hair in a simple, shining wedge cut, a style she adopted in high school and intends to keep. When we eat lunch together between presentations, she displays precise, neat, fastidious habits; Julie would never dribble salad dressing down her front.

It is not a surprise that Julie has come to the conference. She fits the profile of a newly emerging health consumer: solidly upper to middle class, college educated, well informed, a patient who is aware of and uses some complementary health products and practices, including supplements and chiropractic—none of which she reports to her family doctor or the oncologist managing her kidney cancer. She has health insurance but is willing to spend money for care she deems useful and necessary outside that system.

Julie knows it is up to her to get good health care. Her only complaint about her care so far is that everything seems to be about money. She says renal cancer patients all talk about the need for more research, more clinical trials of promising therapies. Her health insurance company presently denies coverage to "experimental therapies," including RCTs endorsed by the National Institutes of Health. Right now, she tells us, her odds of survival are the same as they would have been 30 years ago. If surgery can excise the cancer, renal cancer is curable. But most people are not diagnosed early enough.

*They say my cancer was probably silent and growing for eight or more years before I had any symptoms at all. Most people already have diagnosable metastatic renal cancer before they know anything is wrong. My oncologist finally told me that chances are good that they got most of the cancer, but he can't say I'm cured. There is no diagnostic test or ways to screen for kidney cancer, not yet. My best chance for a cure is to find something using immune system strate-*

*gies—that's why I'm here, and why I'm going to NIH to see if I qualify for an experimental protocol.*

## Coley's Toxins

The "spontaneous remission" of cancer has been observed and documented for centuries. From ancient Egyptian times to the present these disappearances of tumors have often been associated with infectious diseases that produce high fever. The Greek Parmenides declared, "Give me the power to induce fever and I will cure all diseases," and the distinguished seventeenth-century English physician, Sydenham, described fever as "a mighty engine which nature brings into the world for the conquest of her enemies." Over the centuries, malaria, mumps, tuberculosis, and scarlet fever sufferers have all experienced—and their physicians have recorded—the disappearance of palpable tumors.

At the end of the nineteenth century, Dr. William B. Coley, a New York City surgeon just out of Harvard Medical School, began to experiment with inducing infectious disease and high fever in cancer patients to trigger remission. In his own time, Coley experienced much resistance and little acceptance. Today, he is recognized as the father of all immunotherapy.

Coley began his work when he observed a full regression of a large and highly visible cancer of the head and neck after the patient had experienced *erysipelas*, a severe skin infection, and a high fever of many days' duration. Dr. Coley began to experiment with live bacterial injections that were highly dangerous. Subsequently, he discovered that he could more safely use heat-killed bacteria (*Streptococcus pyogenes* and *Serratia marcescens*) to produce similar results.

Without being able to identify it molecularly, Coley was actually using a combination of bacterial proteins that caused the immune system to manufacture T cells with prodigious amounts of powerful cancer-combating molecules called "cytokines." These cytokines included what we now call tumor necrosis factor, the interleukins, and interferon. Coley called the bacterial protein his "active principle."

We know Coley lost patients. Artificially inducing an infection, or even producing a high fever in debilitated patients, can be deadly. He also apparently had spectacular cures, full remissions. The results of a thousand cases, preserved and evaluated retrospectively by a team gathered by Dr. Coley's daughter, Mrs. Helen Coley Nauts, suggest that patients with operable cancer had a 50 percent 5-year survival, while those with inoperable cancer had a 45 percent survival. The best results were in patients with sarcoma, where the 5-year survival was 80 percent, and breast cancer—65 percent in inoperable patients, 100 percent in patients who were operable or had early stage cancer.

Coley's work is duly noted in textbooks of oncology, but only, as DeVita's text tells us, as a catalyst to later efforts to "search for more reliable methods of enhancing anti-tumor immunity." These later efforts have, indeed, been fruitful.

Beginning in the 1950s, scientists, such as Memorial Sloan Kettering's Dr. Lloyd Old, have used BCG (Bacillus Calmette-Guerin)—a killed form of tuberculosis bacteria—to stimulate the immune response and produce remissions of melanomas, leukemias, and bladder cancer. Subsequently, recombinant DNA technology has been used to create interleukins and interferons, which have sometimes worked very well, especially against chronic myelogenous leukemia and hairy cell leukemia. Most recently, monoclonal antibodies against specific cancer cell antigens have been designed.

These modern therapies, particularly the interferons and interleukins, are now easy to create and measure, but they tend to be toxic. And so far they have not proven nearly as effective as their researchers had hoped. Meanwhile, other investigators have continued to follow in William Coley's footsteps.

In his summary of Dr. Coley's work at Comprehensive Cancer Care, Dr. Ralf Kleef, who did his postdoctoral work at Memorial Sloan-Kettering with Dr. Lloyd Old, reminded us that Dr. Coley's cure rates became lower over time. He and others have theorized that the effects of Coley's nineteenth-century toxins were diluted in a heavily vaccinated twentieth-century population that had few, if any, prior severe, febrile illnesses. His mixed bacterial toxins, they believe, were more effective in those whose immune systems had received and successfully responded to prior infections.

All this led Dr. Kleef and other investigators—and us—to wonder if there might not be other ways to successfully mobilize, as Coley did, the whole panoply of cytokines that fever provokes; to engage the full spectrum of the immune system's natural healing capacity. The other immunomodulating therapies presented at the 1998 Comprehensive Cancer Care conference reflect this hope. One uses a cancer vaccine, MTH–68/H, and the other a biologically active substance found in mistletoe.

## MTH–68/H

Dr. Alan Freeman, of Hadassah Hospital in Jerusalem, reported data on early clinical trials using a vaccine developed in Hungary by Dr. Laszlo Csatary from the Newcastle Disease Virus (NDV), which had been first studied in the early 1960s. Dr. Csatary was ill, so his work was presented at the Comprehensive Cancer Care conference by his colleague, Dr. Tibor Bakacs.

Interested in accounts of cancer regressions after viral infections, Dr. Csatary first noted the powerful anti-cancer effect of the NDV virus in the 1960s. He had observed that during an epidemic of NDV among a Hungarian poultry farmer's chickens, the farmer had had a remarkable regression of a metastatic gastric carcinoma.

The NDV virus the farmer contracted causes respiratory and neurological disease in chickens and is an RNA virus. This means it has no DNA of its own, but must infiltrate the DNA of another cell before it can replicate. NDV does not, as far as is known, cause disease in humans, although occasionally it may provoke cases of conjunctivitis. What NDV does do, in studies in laboratory cancer cell lines and in mice, is induce cancer cell death.

In Dr. Csatary's and Dr. Freeman's experiments, NDV invades cancer cells—but not normal cells—and causes lysis, or destruction of these cells. It also has a general immune-enhancing effect, perhaps, like Coley's toxins, inducing lymphocytes to produce large amounts of cytokines, including interleukin, interferon, and tumor necrosis factor. The NDV virus also appears to possess some other anti-tumor activity because it can cause tumor regression in mice that have severely compromised immune systems.

The MTH–68/H strain of the vaccine that Dr. Freeman worked with in his experimental trials in Israel was developed by Dr. Csatary and previously used in animal and human studies. In one experiment, injections of MTH–68/H caused permanent regression of tumors in 17 of 18 mice; another study by Csatary and his colleagues showed amelioration of symptoms and/or regression of tumors in 4 patients with advanced carcinoma. A third experiment established that the dose of the virus was critical to its effectiveness. These dose-specific, significant tumor responses encouraged Dr. Freeman. He obtained the MTH–68/H vaccine and treated 4 children with brain tumors.

Three of Dr. Freeman's patients had high-grade glioblastomas, tumors that have almost 100 percent mortality and a life expectancy of less than a year. The fourth had an equally virulent but rare and slightly different tumor, gliomatosis cerebri. All had received and exhausted conventional therapies before they came to Dr. Freeman. The parents of these children agreed to the experimental MTH–68/H treatment because they had no good alternatives and they were convinced it was a promising, though unproven, treatment.

All four patients were given MTH–68/H. The 11-year-old girl with gliomatosis cerebri did not do well. After conventional treatment, she had had a 2-month remission before the tumor returned. She received MTH–68/H beginning in March 1997. By August, she had begun to deteriorate, and she died in December. Although she is classified as a "non-responder," she did have a longer period of response to MTH–68/H than she had to standard treatment.

The responses in the other three cases were significant enough to suggest—to the Comprehensive Cancer Care commentator and to us—that MTH–68/H should continue to be studied in larger clinical trials. In two cases, the children on MTH–68/H show stable disease: The tumors are not shrinking, but also are not growing. Neurologically and physically, the children are functioning well.

The third child, now a young teenager, began treatment with MTH–68/H in May 1996. He was, Dr. Freeman says, in "terrible condition" after standard treatment. He was functioning poorly, in a wheelchair, convulsing. His life expectancy was a few weeks, a couple of months at most.

After he started treatment, symptomatic improvement was noted very quickly. The tumor did not shrink at first, but then began, slowly and steadily, to decrease in size; after 18 months it was about 70 percent smaller. The boy is now off all medication—including antiseizure drugs—except the viral vaccine, which he receives every day. He is in school now and is reportedly a very good student.

Dr. Freeman introduced this patient, who was present at the Comprehensive Cancer Care conference with his parents. The self-conscious adolescent stood, looking perfectly normal, and reacting as any teenager would in this situation: He clearly would rather have been somewhere else, certainly not in a room full of adults who were all staring at him, grinning, and applauding. His parents, understandably, were delighted.

Dr. Freeman says this is not alternative therapy, but "pre-conventional therapy . . . (to be studied) in a very rigid fashion. We need," he went on, "to evaluate how it works, at a molecular level, and what immune mechanisms it evokes." MTH–68/H is currently being investigated in clinical trials in Europe and Israel. No trials are available in the United States. We hope this will change. This seems to us exactly the kind of situation that cries out for more research: tumors with grim prognoses; no effective conventional treatment; and a promising, nontoxic approach.

## Mistletoe

Dr. Josef Beuth, the president of the German Society of Oncology, has published widely on both conventional and alternative cancer therapies. He works with a group at the University of Cologne and has been studying European mistletoe (*Viscum album*) in the laboratory and in clinical trials for 10 years. Before he discussed his research data at Comprehensive Cancer Care, he offered a brief history of the therapeutic use of mistletoe.

Mistletoe has had a long history of folk use in religious ceremonies and in healing in Europe. It was only in 1920, however, that the German biologist and spiritual teacher Rudolf Steiner proposed that the plant could be used in cancer treatment. Since then, physicians who adhere to Steiner's "anthroposophical" teachings, and other scientists, have tested this therapy—in a variety of formulations—and explored its effectiveness.

In 1989 two German scientists isolated an immunoactive component, "mistletoe lectin one," from the standardized extract, which is called "Iscador." Lectins are glycoproteins, combinations of carbohydrate and protein. One chain, or component, of mistletoe, "lectin one" is cytotoxic (able to cause cancer cell death), and the other, "lectin two," has the specific "lectin" activity, the capacity to bind cancer-destroying T cells to a tumor cell receptor. Mistletoe is also a strong nonspecific immune activator, apparently significantly increasing levels of several interleukins as well as tumor necrosis factor–alpha.

Animal studies have shown that mistletoe encourages proliferation of immune cells, protects the immune system from destruction by cytotoxic drugs, and inhibits the growth of primary tumors and the spread of metastases. In one study on an experimentally induced sarcoma, 90 percent of the control animals died while 80 percent of those treated with mistletoe lived. In early, noncontrolled, human clinical trials with 200 patients, mistletoe extract produced a significant increase in blood immune cells and a rise in endorphin production and enhanced the quality of life of patients who took it. It appeared to investigators that the lectin acted not only to increase immune response but also to promote a wider biological stimulation.

Randomized clinical trials so far (with patients with glioblastoma and advanced colon cancer) continue to confirm that the mistletoe lectin has the ability to stimulate the immune system, increase endorphin levels, and enhance quality of life. These findings suggest that mistletoe is a powerful treatment capable, like the Chinese herbal therapies discussed in Chapter 6, of enhancing immune response and improving patient comfort level on its own; as a complement to conventional therapies; or as part of a comprehensive, integrative treatment. We would like, along with Dr. Beuth, to add that mistletoe should be taken under medical supervision. It may on occasion increase blood pressure and heart rate. It should definitely not be used by anyone taking monoamine oxidase inhibitor antidepressants, with which it interacts.

## Julie's Search Continues

Julie came to the Comprehensive Cancer Care knowing conventional biomedicine had done its best job by removing her cancerous kidney. She and her oncologist had already agreed that radiation and chemotherapy, although used for her stage and type of cancer, demonstrated little advantage either for extending her life or preventing any metastases. The scientific data simply didn't convince either of them that the risks of aggressive therapy were balanced by any possible benefit to Julie.

At the Comprehensive Cancer Care conference, Julie filled notebooks with suggested therapeutic interventions that might strengthen her immune system. The fact that many of these were long-term strategies—the dietary changes and herbs and mind-body techniques that were directed at improving her health over time— was both heartening and amusing to her. *I've been a planner all my life. I believe present action guides future outcomes. The worst thing about cancer was how hopeless and helpless I felt, and how dependent I was on things I didn't control and didn't understand. I've always been healthy, and I've always been conservative and cautious. Now I have a sense of what I need to do.*

Because she knew that kidney cancer was particularly responsive to immune enhancement, Julie resolved to begin a regimen consisting of the dietary changes we recommend in Chapter 5 and the phytonutrients we discuss in Chapter 8. She also decided to find a mind-body skills group in her area. And, after the sessions on immune modulatory therapies, she was excited about the possibility of using a well-researched therapy specifically designed to stimulate her immune system.

Julie was impressed with the data on Coley's toxins but was uneasy about trying the hyperthermia treatments she had only heard about on the Internet. The information on MTH–68/H was impressive to her, but trials were not underway in the United States and she wasn't ready to leave her young family and go to Hungary or Israel.

By the time the Comprehensive Cancer Care conference was over, Julie had decided she would either start on mistletoe—the evidence had looked good to her—or begin a course of Chinese herbal therapy. She would go home and see which qualified and experienced practitioners of both approaches were most accessible to her.

Julie remained undecided about signing on for the NIH experimental protocol. From the beginning, she had tried to make choices based on her conservative instincts; she wanted to proceed warily and do the least harmful treatments first. She felt slightly guilty that she was not ready to be part of an experiment that might benefit future patients. Maybe at some point, but not now.

Julie had been, she said, inclined to think of life as good and evil, black and white, on or off. It had not occurred to her, when she was first diagnosed, that effective treatment might involve several different modalities and might not focus entirely on eliminating cancer cells. Listening to various clinicians talk about combination therapies, considering ways she could enhance her inherent capacity for self-healing, she began to see her cancer as presenting multiple possibilities for control. In her situation, she told us, it made sense to worry less about tumor growth and think more about mobilizing her immune system to protect her.

# 8

# Nature's Pharmacy: Phytonutrients and Nutraceuticals

THE THERAPEUTIC SUBSTANCES we discuss in this chapter—shark cartilage, Essiac tea, Hoxsey's Formula, mushrooms, Coenzyme Q10, melatonin, and green tea—are naturally occurring compounds that have the ability to modulate biologic activity in the body. They are parts of animals or plants or can be isolated from them. Most of these substances have known, documented pharmaceutical actions: They act on the cells, tissues, and organs and have measurable and predictable effects. These compounds are sometimes called phytochemicals or nutraceuticals. Many have a long history of human use as natural medicines for cancer, as well as other conditions, and some have received wide public attention in popular books or promotions by advocates. These biological modulators were presented by researchers at the Comprehensive Cancer Care conferences in 1998 and 1999 and most are now being tested in clinical trials.

Until the last few years, most of the research on these substances was done in countries other than the United States. There were cultural and ideological barriers in the United States to the study of traditional, folk, herbal, or unconventional remedies. They were treated, often with derision, as "old wives' tales." When extravagant and unverified claims were made for the therapies—and the contents were treated as closely guarded secrets—they were regarded with far more skepticism, even by many people interested in alternative and complementary therapies, including us. When they were heavily promoted, and costly, they were widely condemned as charlatanism and quackery.

Equally important, there were economic obstacles to studying these remedies. Almost by definition, nutraceuticals are substances that are commonly available in nature and difficult to patent. Manufacturers are unwilling to fund expensive research into remedies that do not offer opportunities to make large profits.

The situation, however, is changing. The more closely and respectfully we look at the world's healing traditions, the more interested the practitioners have become in remedies that seem to have stood the test of time. Because half of all cancer patients still fail to respond to conventional treatment or experience later recurrence of their primary tumor, and because Congress has mandated money for the study of complementary and alternative therapies, significant numbers of highly qualified researchers—and corporations—are now beginning to investigate these treatments.

The creation and funding of NIH's Office of Alternative Medicine (OAM) in 1991 opened the door. The transformation of the office into the more fully funded National Center for Complementary and Alternative Medicine (NCCAM), and the creation in 1998 by the NCI of an Office of Cancer Complementary and Alternative Medicine (OCCAM), have paved the way for a more systematic approach to studying these therapies and more funding to undertake these studies. The work presented at CCC I and II reflects both the longstanding worldwide interest in using and evaluating natural remedies and more recent U.S. efforts to explore and document their possible value in cancer care.

## Shark Cartilage

In the last few years, we have seen many stories on the promise of drugs that act to inhibit "angiogenesis," or blood vessel formation.

To grow beyond 1 to 2 millimeters—pinhead size—solid tumors must develop new circulation. Angiogenesis is the process by which tumors induce cells from mature capillaries to grow at an abnormally rapid rate, forming new capillaries that connect the tumor to the circulating blood supply. These new capillaries bring nourishment to the tumor and also open a pathway to metastasis, the spread of the cancer from its original site.

If solid tumors need a new circulation to grow and metastasize, then it stands to reason that interfering with the growth of these new capillaries can frustrate both the spread of the tumor and its growth at its original site. Agents that accomplish this are described as "antiangiogenic."

The scientific establishment, preoccupied with ways of killing tumor cells, has paid little attention to antiangiogenic substances until quite recently. In the last several years, however, Dr. Judah Folkman, who did some of the earliest research on angiogenesis in cancer, has been widely recognized for discerning and developing antiangiogenic compounds. At the same time, a number of scientists have begun to explore the antiangiogenic power of cartilage, which seems to inhibit both angiogenesis and cancer invasion.

The first research on cartilage in the United States was undertaken in 1958 when Dr. John Prudden of Columbia University began to investigate the potential of bovine (cow) tracheal cartilage for accelerating post-surgical wound healing. By the early 1970s Prudden was using bovine cartilage to treat tumors and reporting on both partial and complete responses in many patients with advanced cancer. Research by Prudden and others confirmed that cartilage could prevent angiogenesis as well as stimulate immunity and inhibit the protease activity that contributes to tumor invasiveness.

Research on shark cartilage followed in the 1980s, first on tumors implanted in the eyes of rabbits and then on human melanomas transplanted into mice bred specifically for cancer research. The first studies showed that the tumors in mice given shark cartilage shrank, whereas those in controls grew extremely fast.

Clinical testing of shark cartilage done in Cuba in 1992 was subsequently reported on national television (*60 Minutes,* February and

July 1993). Although this trial wasn't presented in a peer-reviewed journal, the public interest in and response to the TV coverage was immense. The Cuban study was designed to assess the safety and effectiveness of high doses of powdered shark cartilage. This trial involved 29 patients with various advanced-stage cancers: prostate (2), central nervous system (5), ovarian (2), uterine (2), stomach (2), esophageal (2), tonsil (2), liver (2), and bladder (1). The patients were given 1 to 2.25 grams of shark cartilage per kilogram of body weight daily (in rectal enemas) for the first 6 weeks and the same dosage orally for 10 additional weeks.

At the conclusion of the trial, tumor size reductions were recorded for prostate tumors (15–67 percent), ovarian tumors (15–25 percent), and breast tumors (up to 50 percent). Central nervous system tumors showed no growth. Eight patients died during the study. Twenty-one were still alive 30 weeks after the trial ended.

Detailed autopsies were done on 5 patients. Evaluations of the tumors showed changes in the vasculature and encapsulation of tumor tissue. Deep fibrotic tissue surrounding the tumors and necrosis (cell death) in the tumor itself were observed. These changes, verified by tissue examination by outside experts, appeared to confirm that shark cartilage modified the development of new blood vessels and stimulated fibrotic action and necrosis of tumors.

Charles Simone, M.D., visited Cuba during the trial and examined patients at 6, 16, and 20 weeks into the study. Since then, Dr. Simone has continued clinical trials on the use of shark cartilage in cancer. At the Comprehensive Cancer Care conference in 1998, Dr. Simone summarized early results: In 35 patients who had no response to any previous conventional treatment, the response rate was 12 out of 35, or 34 percent.

Shark cartilage seems to act by stopping the tumor signals that trigger capillary growth and by keeping intact the intervening cell walls, which can frustrate the growth and connection of these capillaries to the tumor. Instead of killing the cancer cells—and other dividing cells that may be healthy—shark cartilage cuts off the supply lines, maintains the integrity of the cell walls, and places the tumor in a no-growth zone. For the tumor, whose job is to multiply and proliferate, stability is like death. The cancer is controlled, stopped from development. The cancer cells eventually die, as was seen during the autopsies done during this study.

Shark cartilage was originally, and is still usually, administered by mouth in powder form. Recent studies, including the work in Cuba, have suggested that doses far larger than customarily used—120 grams versus 15 grams—may be significantly more effective. These studies also suggest that administration by a rectal retention enema may be more effective and better tolerated by patients who object to the odor and the taste of the powder. Shark cartilage, although occasionally causing mild nausea or diarrhea, has been shown to be nontoxic in both animal and human studies. It is classified as a food—a nutritional substance—and can be legally sold over the counter under the 1994 law regulating the marketing of supplements.

In practice, many doctors prescribing complementary medical treatment for cancer have found that administration of large doses of shark cartilage appears to be effective for some cancer patients in controlling cancer growth and even causing regression of tumors. Although there are as yet no results from controlled studies, practitioners, and many more patients acting on their own, use the cartilage in conjunction with a wide range of other conventional and complementary therapies.

The FDA-approved trials of shark cartilage presently being pursued will help to establish its efficacy and determine future testing and uses. At CCC I, we learned that three FDA-approved Phase II trials on Stage IV patients, using shark cartilage as the only therapy, were underway. Two are being done in northern New Jersey and one in Chicago at Northwestern University. This kind of protocol should provide more information on the efficacy of shark cartilage. Because shark cartilage does not usually cause rapid, measurable tumor shrinkage, a "good" response will be cessation or slowing of tumor growth and/or an inhibition of metastases. And, if this response persists, the use of shark cartilage in the treatment of certain cancers should proceed to more extensive, Phase III clinical trials.

## Hoxsey's Formula and Essiac Tea

Hoxsey's Formula and Essiac tea were both developed early in this century and are still marketed as "cancer cures" today. Hoxsey's Formula is a compound of several different herbs found in the United States that are extracted and combined in solution. It is used in the United States and Mexico. Essiac tea is widely available and used, especially in Canada. The Canadian government is presently studying these herbal formulas, in carefully designed, "blinded" trials.

Essiac tea has been promoted as an Ojibway Indian cure for cancer since 1922. The Canadian nurse who made it popular, Renée Caisse (Essiac in reverse) claimed she was given the formula by a local Native American healer who was a member of the Ojibway tribe. Anti-tumor activity for some of the individual herbs—slippery elm, burdock root, Indian rhubarb, and sorrel—has been reported, but tests by the NCI in 1983 found that the combination had no activity in reducing animal tumors. No severe side effects have been reported in using Essiac tea.

Flor-Essence is reportedly a version of Essiac that Ms. Caisse was working on before her death. It contains the herbs mentioned above, plus blessed thistle, watercress, kelp, and red clover blossom. The company producing this product is currently conducting more rigorous studies.

The Hoxsey Formula, developed by Harry Hoxsey in the early 1920s, contains a mixture of 8 herbs and also is part of an external remedy for skin tumors. The major components of the Hoxsey internal formula are cascara, potassium iodide, red clover, buckthorn bark, burdock root, licorice root, prickly ash bark, stillingia root, berberis root, and pokeberries and poke root. Some of these herbs have known biological actions. Licorice, as we've mentioned, has anti-tumor and immune-stimulating activity, and red clover contains genistein (as does soy), which inhibits angiogenesis and provokes tumor cell death. Advocates of this remedy suggest, as well, that the particular combination is more powerful than the single herbs listed.

At first, Hoxsey sought to keep his formula secret, as proprietary information, but his encounters with the legal system required him to reveal the contents. Hoxsey also continued to modify the contents, sometimes omitting cascara (a bowel stimulant some find too strong) or adjusting the proportions of the herbal doses.

Dr. James A. Duke, who is one of the world's recognized authorities on herbs and their medicinal use, pointed out at CCC I that both Hoxsey's Formula and Essiac tea contained burdock and red clover, both of which have a long history of use in Native American culture and by this continent's European settlers. Dr. Duke reported that in laboratory testing both burdock and red clover exhibited strong anti-inflammatory effects and have shown anti-carcinogenic action in some experiments on cancer cell lines. Dr. Duke believes that these herbs have useful, supportive action in treating chronic degenerative conditions and might indeed be useful in treating cancer.

We have talked over the years to a number of people with cancer who have found one or the other formula helpful. They report feeling better, having more energy, increased appetite, and less pain—no small gains in the life of a cancer patient. However, these reports do not establish Hoxsey's Formula or Essiac tea as a first-line or sole treatment for cancer. Nor do we know if the combinations of herbs in the Hoxsey and Essiac products have any synergistic effect, such as those we've seen in Chinese herbal combinations.

We know these formulas have been around a long time; that they contain active anti-cancer herbs, and that they are, if used in moderation, nontoxic. We believe they may be helpful as part of an integrated treatment, but we do not yet know how much or for whom. We know people will continue to use these remedies, based on anecdotes and even folklore. The choice to do so should be made by people fully aware of the lack of documented evidence. The Canadian studies now being done will help establish whether or not there is a basis for continued research.

## The Therapeutic Use of Mushrooms: *Maitake-D*

In many healing traditions, mushrooms are recognized as a powerful source of physiologically active substances. They have been used in Asia for centuries as a remedy for infections and cancer. Chinese *ganoderma* mushroom (called *Reishi* by the Japanese), for example, has long been prized for its immune-enhancing effect. We also know that psychoactive mushrooms have been used for millennia for spiritual purposes in many cultures. Now, researchers are reporting that the mushrooms many of us include in our diets have a place in cancer treatment.

In the 1970s, researchers in Asia began to extract and isolate biologically active polysaccharides with anti-cancer effects from common mushrooms, including shiitake and *Maitake*. By 1977, the Japanese had isolated three biological response modifiers that were approved by the Japanese Food and Drug Administration for cancer treatment. In 1992, the U.S. National Cancer Institute began to study extracts and active fractions from the *Maitake* mushroom.

At the 1999 Comprehensive Cancer Care conference Dr. Cun Zhuang presented research on one fraction of one of these mushrooms: *Maitake-D*. Born in China, educated in both China and Japan, Dr. Cun is a biochemist who is particularly concerned with bioactive substances present in both mushrooms and seaweed. He came to the United States in the 1970s and continued his work on the active polysaccharides he found in these food products.

*Maitake-D* has more recently been the subject of intensive animal studies, both in Japan and in the United States. According to Dr. Cun, in one study complete tumor remission was experienced in 80 percent of cancer-induced animals fed *Maitake-D*. Of all the mushroom extracts, *Matiake-D* has consistently shown the strongest effect. This extract has exhibited potent activity, inhibiting both carcinogenesis (initiation of cancer) and metastasis. The animal research suggests that *Maitake-D* increases the body's ability to kill tumors by activating the immune system. *Maitake-D* stimulates both natural killer cell activity and production of interleukin-1.

Dr. Cun also presented clinical studies and case reports that demonstrate *Maitake-D's* effectiveness in cancer of the breast, lung, liver, prostate, and brain. Used with chemotherapy, it allows lower effective dosage, with less toxicity and far fewer side effects.

As a postscript, Dr. Cun mentioned that, in the United States, natural, nontoxic therapies have largely been studied in very advanced cancers. Like many researchers and patients, he would like to see these substances used earlier in treatment, as a first line, rather than a last line, of defense against cancer.

## Green Tea

In recent years, the search for agents capable of preventing or suppressing cancer growth has been stimulated by epidemiological studies that correlate cancer rates and the consumption of certain foods and beverages. One of the most striking correlations has been between the consumption of green tea (*Camellia sinesis*) and the rate of cancer.

In the early 1980s researchers in the United States and Japan had begun to wonder why heavy smokers in Japan had only one-third the rate of lung cancer as those in the United States. Eventually they realized one important difference was the amount of green tea that the Japanese consumed. In time, they isolated an active factor in green tea, a polyphenol called epigallocatechin, which, they believed, engendered this chemopreventive (use of a specific substance to prevent a particular disease) effect.

Tea is the most widely consumed beverage in the world. Green tea, black tea, and oolong are the three commercially sold varieties. Most of the current studies focus on green tea, but a few studies suggest that the biologically active factors—the polyphenols, like epigallocatechin—may be available in all forms. Research shows that these polyphenols:

- Act as antioxidants, both by scavenging damaging free radicals and by enhancing enzyme activities that contribute to DNA repair.
- Protect the skin from carcinogenic damage from solar radiation and exposure to chemicals (in animal models).
- Exert a significant protective effect on both the development and severity of tumors induced in the stomachs and esophagi of mice.
- Act (in animal testing) to decrease the carcinogenic effect of heterocyclic animes (HCAs) formed by grilling or

frying meat. (HCAs are thought to be associated with cancers of the breast, colon, and pancreas in meat-eating populations.)

- Help maintain stable white blood cell counts (WBCs) in patients undergoing chemotherapy.
- Exercise a chemoprotective effect on women with breast cancer manifested by decreasing recurrence rates and numbers of positive lymph nodes and increasing disease-free survival.

Green tea, with glowing reports of chemoprevention and treatment activity, and few toxic side effects, is as close to a perfect phytonutrient as we've seen. Virtually all those who offer comprehensive care now recommend the inclusion of green tea as part of an anti-cancer strategy and as a chemopreventive agent. More human studies are being done to assess the mechanism of action, optimum dose, and range of effects. Right now, the data suggest that anyone can benefit by drinking green tea daily to promote healthy immune system functioning or as part of a cancer treatment plan.

## Coenzyme Q10

Coenzyme Q10 is a vitaminlike substance that is present in the cells of all mammals and plays an important role in the cell's energy-producing mitochondria. It is a potent antioxidant and its declining tissue concentration may contribute to the aging process and to the progress of degenerative diseases. Because the heart has very high metabolic activity, it requires large amounts of CoQ10. In Japan, CoQ10 is routinely used as a treatment in cardiac care, particularly for congestive heart failure and cardiomyopathy. In studies done in Europe, CoQ10 has been used to successfully reduce chemotherapy-induced heart damage. More recently, it has been studied as a significant part of cancer treatment, as an antioxidant agent that may affect tumor growth in cancer patients.

At the Comprehensive Cancer Care conference, Dr. Richard Willis of the University of Texas reported on work done by himself and by

Dr. Carl Folkers, among others. In one remarkable uncontrolled clinical study, done in Denmark, 32 node-positive breast cancer patients were treated with conventional therapy and with 90 mg per day of CoQ10 plus other supplements. All these patients survived at least 24 months, a period of time in which it was expected that 6 would die. Partial tumor regression was observed in 6 patients. Two of these people were later given 300 to 400 mg of CoQ10 a day, and complete remissions followed. Several more studies on individual patients were done using similarly high doses of CoQ10, with similar results.

These results may be due partly to the antioxidant effect of CoQ10, or perhaps to an immune-enhancing effect to which recent research points. There is no evidence to indicate that CoQ10 interferes with conventional treatment; indeed, it has been successfully used to mitigate the cardiotoxicity of chemotherapy. No toxicity has been observed using CoQ10 itself, even at very high doses.

As Dr. Willis said, the data are promising, and the investigation continues, but only case studies have been published. Randomized clinical trials have not been completed. The evidence available is strong enough so that some clinicians and many patients are using CoQ10 as an adjunctive therapy. We recommend it as well.

## Melatonin

Melatonin, a hormone produced by the pineal gland, has become popular as a nontoxic remedy for jet lag and insomnia. In our tissues, the melatonin levels fluctuate daily, rising at night and decreasing during the day, as a response to available light. In epidemiological studies, low levels of circulating melatonin are found in people with sleep disturbances and in some patients with chronic disease, including cancer. Some circumstantial evidence in studies of mice have suggested a link between levels of artificially administered nocturnal light, which depresses melatonin production, and some cancers.

Melatonin acts as an antioxidant, both as a potent scavenger of free radicals and as a stimulant of the main antioxidant enzyme of the brain, glutathione peroxidase. Melatonin is diffused through all the tissues of the body, including intracellular membranes. As a widely available antioxidant, it provides broad protective action against DNA damage by free radicals.

Recently, investigators have discovered that melatonin inhibits the proliferation of some cancer cell lines in the laboratory and slows the growth of a large number of induced cancers in mice. Other studies show that melatonin demonstrates a direct inhibitory effect on estrogen-responsive cells. This antiestrogenic activity had optimal effects when dosage was available on a diurnal schedule, corresponding to the natural secretion of melatonin by the pineal gland.

Melatonin levels are commonly abnormal in cancer patients. The nighttime rise in melatonin has been found to be suppressed in some women with breast cancer and to be absent or depressed in men with prostate cancer. One study tested the relationship between immune response and melatonin production, finding that administering the immune factor interleukin-2 to patients restored normal melatonin levels and the diurnal rhythm of secretion.

Stress is known as a suppressor of both melatonin and the immune system, suggesting a biochemical relationship between this particular hormone and the immune system. And in one fascinating study by Dr. Ann Massion and her colleagues at the University of Massachusetts, daily meditation was found to increase levels of melatonin in healthy women.

At the 1999 Comprehensive Cancer Care conference, David Blask, Ph.D., senior research associate at the Bassett Research Institute in Cooperstown, New York, discussed the use of melatonin with tamoxifen. Tamoxifen, which is recommended for preventive treatment in breast cancer patients, has several troubling side effects, including increased risk of uterine cancer. Many patients also develop a resistance to the antiestrogenic effects of tamoxifen.

According to Dr. Blask's work, melatonin increases the effectiveness of tamoxifen, up to 100 times in laboratory testing, in inhibiting the proliferation of breast cancer cells. This suggests that melatonin supplementation may make it possible to use lower and less toxic doses of tamoxifen. This should reduce the risk of uterine cancers and lower the chance of developing tamoxifen resistance. Dr. Blask regards this research as a good example of integrative cancer care: using conventional care with complementary medicine. We agree; and so do the many researchers who are studying ways to use combinations of therapeutic agents to reduce toxicity, and increase efficacy.

Other research on melatonin alone or in combination with other treatments is equally interesting. In Italy, Dr. Paolo Lissoni and his colleagues used melatonin as part of cancer treatment and have published the following results:

- Fifty patients with cancer metastatic to the brain were given either steroids and anticonvulsants alone or in combination with melatonin. The 1-year survival rate was higher in patients who received melatonin.
- Twenty-four patients with solid tumors were given melatonin with interleukin-2. A partial tumor response occurred in 3 patients (12 percent), and 14 patients (59 percent) had stabilized tumor growth.
- Of 40 patients with advanced melanoma given melatonin, 6 had partial responses (15 percent) and 6 stabilized (15 percent).
- Of 20 patients with non-small cell lung cancer given melatonin plus interleukin-2, 4 had a partial response (20 percent) and 10 stabilized (50 percent).

All of these reports mark melatonin as a substance with promising anti-cancer activity, no reported toxicity, and a capacity to work independently and as an adjunct to conventional therapy. These studies, and laboratory testing done in the United States, suggest that melatonin also seems to be one of those agents that acts by multiple mechanisms. It stimulates the immune system, reduces circulating hormones (such as estrogen) that promote tumor progression, induces differentiation in cancer cells, inhibits angiogenesis, and inhibits metastasis.

Although melatonin has low toxicity, it is a hormone that may have long-term negative effects in some people. In particular, there are studies indicating that it may be contraindicated in people with leukemia. More generally, and emphatically, we suggest that all long-term use of melatonin as a part of cancer care should be medically supervised.

We expect, as Dr. Blask suggested, that this naturally occurring hormone will be carefully explored as we search for less toxic therapies. In fact, a radiation oncologist who attended CCC II, Dr. Lawrence Birk, has already begun to design a multisite study of melatonin as an adjunct to radiation treatment of brain metastases.

We hope that soon melatonin and some of the other demonstrably effective phytochemicals will be thoughtfully studied, not only as adjuncts to therapy for advanced disease but also as part of comprehensive programs of care for early stage cancer; as chemopreventative agents; and even, where appropriate, in comparison to more conventional treatments that lack curative power.

Meanwhile, hopeful and desperate cancer patients will continue to try these substances based on information gathered from many sources. We have encouraged patients to be aware of the research and to explore their use with their doctors as promising adjunctive therapies (e.g., tamoxifen used with melatonin), and we strongly suggest that health professionals learn, as we all must, to be less quick to condemn a therapy just because it seems old-fashioned.

# 9

# Prostate and Breast Cancers

THIS IS THE only chapter entirely devoted to specific kinds of cancers. We do this partly because breast cancer and prostate cancer are extremely common malignancies: In 1999 it was estimated that nearly 180,000 men were diagnosed with prostate cancer and over 176,000 women were told they had breast cancer; during that year 43,000 women died from their disease, and 40,000 men died from metastatic prostate cancer. We also address these cancers separately because of the psychological challenge these conditions bring; because of their prevalence in the rapidly growing age group of 40- to 60-year-olds; and because of the enormous public and research focus on the prevention, detection, and treatment of these conditions.

Women's breasts are an integral part of their personal and sexual identity as well as organs of nursing. They may evoke pleasure, pride, tenderness, and shame. Surgical and medical intervention may produce permanent and irreversible changes in a woman's breasts and in her sense of who she is. The prostate is also intimately connected with sexual functioning. Surgery, radiation, and hormonal treatment may all result in impotence, and surgical intervention often produces incontinence as well, conditions that are devastating emotionally as well as physically. Screening for these cancers triggers fear in almost everyone. Misdiagnoses and misinterpretations of data are common.

## Steve and Grace

Steve and Grace came to the CCC in 1998 because their youngest daughter insisted. Her parents, Ellen told us, had experienced a double tragedy in the previous year. First Grace was diagnosed with breast cancer. Six months later, Steve was told he had prostate cancer.

The statistics on breast and prostate cancer suggest more couples may face this devastating news. And the unexpected and added burden a double cancer diagnosis can place on a family calls for even more careful attention.

Grace, like most women, discovered a lump in her breast almost accidentally. She was in her early fifties, was scheduling mammograms every two years, and had no known risk factors for breast cancer. She examined her breasts "every now and then" but relied on the good habits of a lifetime and a family history free of breast cancer as her best defense against cancer. The rush, from finding a lump through diagnostic tests and consultations with specialists, left her disoriented and confused.

Steve now says he just wanted reassurance: He was 55, he was healthy, and both he and Grace were stunned by her diagnosis. Now they are both living with cancer, trying to make difficult choices. Sometimes they find themselves divided rather than united by their common disease.

Although painful, perhaps the distance they feel from one another is not surprising. Cancer is a life-threatening illness with an uncertain prognosis and often devastating treatments. And, of course, Steve and Grace faced possibly mutilating surgery and threats not only to longevity but to their self-image, their sense of who they were and of how they felt and performed as a man and a woman.

Steve and Grace are quick to deny any real threat to their marriage of 35 years, but their children insist otherwise. Ellen says the cancer undermined more than her parents' health and well-being. Cancer shook every aspect of their comfortable, somewhat complacent life.

Her parents have always been a team, Ellen says. They own a small successful business. They work and play together. The business, their family, and the community life in their small Midwestern city keep them busy. They had few disagreements and fewer conflicts, moving in tandem through the contours of the life they shared. In fact, Ellen reports, she wasn't too surprised when her father told her he had prostate cancer 6 months after the shock of her mother's diagnosis. After all, in the minds of their children and community, Steve and Grace did everything together.

Cancer, as we know, has a way of precipitating both questions and possibilities. Gender differences, differences in coping styles and expectations, and individual experiences in the health system spotlighted small cracks in Steve and Grace's united front. They felt as troubled by the changes in their relationship as they did by the overriding problems of choosing appropriate cancer care, and far less supported in their efforts to deal with these changes.

Grace felt she was unable to tell Steve how frightened she was, or ask him for support. She knew he was worried, and she believed he loved her, but his obvious discomfort only made her withdraw. *I thought, maybe unfairly, that his need for reassurance was becoming oppressive. I turned away. He got more anxious, and I got more resentful.*

Steve was terrified that surgery would make him impotent and incontinent—no longer a man, but a neuter, a baby, in his eyes and Grace's—terrified that without surgery he would die and embarrassed to tell Grace about any of his fears.

After we spent time with this struggling couple, we realized even more clearly how vulnerable and confused people with cancer can feel. The fact that they both had cancer did not help Steve and Grace cope better or feel more supportive or sympathetic. Small differences and realistic fears were magnified in the space of mutual fears and withdrawal, something that probably wouldn't have happened or been so troubling if cancer had been diagnosed in only one of them.

For example, Steve had been adamant about Grace accepting and pursuing the therapy, a radical mastectomy, suggested by the surgeon she first consulted. This doctor had said that in his experience, any eventual recurrence and death from breast cancer was best prevented by fast, complete surgical intervention, followed by aggressive chemotherapy. No other options were offered, and when Grace suggested other possibilities, he dismissed them with a wave of his hand. Grace wanted a second opinion.

Meanwhile, Steve had been terrified. To him, any delay, any possibility of her death, was painful beyond belief. He felt she was rejecting life, and rejecting him, by seeking more information and delaying treatment.

Grace, on the other hand, felt pressured to make her decision on too little evidence, in too little time. She wanted to have her breast as well as her life, and Steve couldn't seem to get it. Explaining this to Steve proved difficult, and she finally just found another doctor recommended by a friend. This second doctor, who practiced at a nearby university hospital, said that her mammogram, her ultrasound, and the results of two biopsies suggested to him that Grace was a good candidate for state-of-the-art breast conservation surgery, followed by radiation.

This threw Steve into even more confusion. He believed Grace was risking her life; she believed she was choosing good mainstream care. She was also discovering other information, on self-care strategies, and found compelling evidence to begin to change her diet, increase her exercise, and join a support group. Steve tried to understand and wanted to be supportive, but he says it was strange stuff, and he was afraid she was becoming a "feminist."

Meanwhile, Grace felt deserted and unsupported. She resented Steve's sarcastic remarks about her choices and felt, for the first time in their marriage, that he was being a typical authoritarian male, belittling her concerns. His alliance with the first doctor—whom she disliked as much for his attitude toward her as a woman as for his arrogant professionalism—made him appear a bully, not a partner. *I resented Steve, and his thoughtlessness, and felt alone. Later, when he was diagnosed, I even had a bad moment thinking, "Now he'll find out what I was going through."*

The thought made her feel guilty and even more withdrawn. Steve knew something was wrong, but his own fears were overwhelming his ability to respond to Grace. They were a close and loving couple, and had been together a long time. When Steve's doctor called and reported his elevated PSA, Steve and Grace admitted that they were both full of resentment. As Steve struggled to absorb the news and ask the right questions, Grace decided they needed more help than the surgeon's knife or their family's prayers.

How could these two, who had been together so long, regain their balance? Ellen says that, as a couple, Steve and Grave had been invincible and that cancer had made them fragile and vulnerable. What one had lacked, the other provided. They were like a tag team.

*But after Dad's diagnosis, they couldn't figure out how to help one another. They both needed so much, and sometimes couldn't see it. Dad wanted to be there for Mom, but he was suffering and resentful. He wasn't ready to admit how scared he was. The prostate cancer shook him to his bones. He was trying to decide what to do, and all the options seemed terrible. Meanwhile, Mom was finding help outside. They just weren't communicating.*

One night, Steve just lost it. He accused Grace of selfishness, of only caring about herself and not caring whether he lived or died. *No one gives me any good options,* he said, *and I think about it every day. Will I live 5, 10, 20 years? Do we have enough insurance, enough money to fight this? Are you going to get worse? How can we be there for one another, when both of us have cancer?*

Grace was shocked. In her view, they were dealing with the same question, cancer, and how to decrease their risk of disease progression or recurrence. Yes, she had joined a group of breast cancer patients and found it very helpful. Yes, she was beginning to take time for herself, for the group, for quiet mornings at home. She knew her chances of remission and was trying to decide whether or not to take tamoxifen. She had to take care of herself and wanted Steve to do the same. *The most important thing in my life is us,* she told Steve. *I want us to be in this together. We're talking about life and death decisions, here. Of course we're both scared and lonely. But we have to do things for ourselves and for each other. They're not separate.*

Steve and Grace sought help from their priest, because for them the church was a natural and neutral ground to discuss their fears about death and illness. They found spiritual comfort and a safe way to talk about Steve's feeling of failure and Grace's need for her support group. Their attendance at Mass, something they did routinely, became a deeper and more thoughtful experience. The ritual was something they could share. Steve says talking with Father Brennan helped them see this moment of crisis as part of their life together, and "cancer" as another important, shared experience offering possibilities and hope.

Slowly, they began to sort out the similarities and the differences in their situations. They realized that they both had early stage disease and that there was time to make well-informed decisions—together. They read about their illnesses and made significant changes in their diet. They started walking together and joined a yoga class. When their daughter Ellen insisted, Steve and Grace decided to attend the 1998 Comprehensive Cancer Care conference. It would be part of their journey. They would stop being isolated victims of cancer and become active and engaged survivors, people living with cancer.

## Prostate Cancer

Prostate cancer risk increases significantly with age. The average patient is 65 years old. The disease is fairly rare in men younger than 50 but almost ubiquitous in older men. According to autopsy reports of American men who died after the age of 80 from other causes, 70–80 percent had asymptomatic and undiagnosed prostate cancer.

Risk factors for prostate cancer, in addition to age, include obesity and a high-fat diet. Risk is also higher in certain groups, including African Americans, as Mike discovered, and men with a positive family history. Signs of possible problems, which may signal benign prostate hypertrophy (BPH) as well as cancer, are manifested by changes in urination (retention, frequency, difficulty starting, and reduced stream, for example) and occasional low back pain. Authorities disagree about when or whether regular PSA testing should be part of routine health planning. The American Cancer Society recommends yearly screening for men over the age of 50. The National Cancer Institute does not. For men over 50 with suggestive symptoms or a family history of cancer, or for those who express high anxiety, we suggest consultation with a qualified urologist and careful examination of the meaning and limitations of testing.

Diagnostic tests include digital rectal exam (DRE), PSA, and transrectal ultrasound (TRUS). An elevated PSA is not a definite sign of prostate cancer. The conventional treatments offered include radical prostatectomy, radiation therapy, and expectant management or watchful waiting. The American Urological Association's (AUA) guidelines require that all these options be offered to patients. However, a report in the journal *Oncology* in 1991 suggests that many physicians continue to treat prostate cancer as aggressively as possible, even when it may adversely affect the patient's quality of life. We also know a number of men who feel they were inadequately informed about options before both surgery and radiation.

In most localized cancers, early detection permits and dictates prompt surgical intervention. In prostate cancer the situation is not so clear. Right now, patients and doctors are making decisions based on incomplete scientific data. The adverse effects of surgical treatment, including impotence and incontinence, can be devastating; the chances of experiencing adverse effects are high (although significantly lower in the hands of experienced surgeons) and the benefits of surgery or radiation are, in some cases, uncertain.

For men over 70 a radical prostatectomy may, indeed, shorten life because the disease progresses slowly. We also don't know for sure whether aggressive treatment of early stage prostate cancer, in younger men, with the risks of complications, has any benefit on longevity or in preventing later cancer progression (although there has been a decrease in overall mortality, probably due to early detection, in recent years). "Nerve sparing" operations by experienced surgeons have, indeed, decreased the risk of impotence and incontinence, but there are many men who, years after the surgery, are furious that they were made "sexual cripples."

One option in selected cases of prostate cancer, the conservative practice of watchful waiting, in the view of some physicians and many patients like Steve, is too passive and even dangerous. Science and technology seem to promise so much. Doctors generally are taught to be active and aggressive, to think in terms of winning or losing. Carefully monitored management is not a clearly defined intervention, yet the research suggests that this option is in certain cases the appropriate one.

In all cases, there is a need for patients to have the most complete information available, for physicians to explore the conventional options and the limit of our scientific knowledge about them, and for physicians and patients to consider appropriate complementary and alternative therapies. All presenters and commentators at the CCC emphasized their belief that many patients with prostate cancer have the time to consider using promising and less-aggressive treatments.

### Listening to Dr. Atkins

Dr. Robert Atkins, who is best known for his low carbohydrate regimen and dietary theories, spoke at the CCC about his experience treating prostate cancer. He spoke not as a researcher with hard evidence but as a clinician with many case histories: almost 200 patients, and a follow-up time of as long as 6 years.

Dr. Atkins described his practice as "true complementary medicine, using a panoply of therapies with different therapeutic effects." He believes that, because prostate cancer is generally slow in developing, it should be managed without aggressive therapy. His first step in the treatment of all patients is hormonal manipulation, a total androgen blockade (with the drug Lupron and other substances) to reduce the tumor mass and lower the PSA. After the initial response, Dr. Atkins withdraws the androgen blockade and then reinstitutes it when PSA levels again rise. Dr. Atkins acknowledges that sexual dysfunction results, but says it is reversible several weeks after the androgen blockade is withdrawn.

At the same time, Dr. Atkins develops an individualized program for each patient, using combinations of various nutrients, herbs, and supplements. The regimen includes many of the substances we have discussed in previous chapters: antioxidants, vitamin E, selenium, essential fatty acids (fish oil, flaxseed oil, gamma linoleic acid, squalene, and conjugated linoleic acid), shark cartilage, Coenzyme Q10, mistletoe extract, and lectins. In addition he uses other "alternative" remedies, including carnivora (an extract of the Venus's flytrap plant) and a variety of herbal formulas. In his presentation, Dr. Atkins pointed out that all of the substances he uses "have been shown in one study or another to contribute to survival, quality of life or extension of life in cancer patients. None are curative, but the entire package can have a powerful effect."

Dr. Atkins believes that 95 percent of his patients are responding to his treatment regimen and that their cancer is under control with few complications. However, the combination of intermittent hormonal therapy, based on levels of PSA, and the individually designed prescription of substances is not a treatment program that is easy to evaluate. Dr. Atkins suggests that the best way to study this kind of multifaceted therapy is to have a treatment center such as his and a conventional cancer center treat a group of carefully matched prostate cancer patients and report the outcomes.

Dr. William Fair, the former chief of Urologic Surgery at Memorial Sloan-Kettering Hospital, was the commentator in this session. Dr. Fair, who is one of the world's experts on the treatment of prostate cancer and a thoughtful proponent of integrative cancer care, began by welcoming Dr. Atkins's research proposal and went on to raise a number of important questions about his presentation.

First, he noted that, because prostate cancer is slow growing, 6 years is not an adequate follow-up and a Dr. Atkins's 95 percent success rate is difficult to evaluate. Next, Dr. Fair discussed some of the limitations of hormonal therapy (which is also used in conventional treatment), including the development of resistance to it and side effects, including anemia, osteoporosis, decreased muscle mass, and fatigue. No form of therapy is universally applicable, Dr. Fair said, and not all prostate cancers are hormonally sensitive. He added that the use of PSA as a tumor marker presented another problem: PSA level does not always indicate tumor volume or aggressiveness.

Steve found Dr. Atkins's information interesting—he didn't know it was safe to combine so many treatment modalities—and he was heartened to think it might be possible to avoid surgery. Dr. Fair's comments were helpful if sobering. Steve began to wonder if it might be possible to use a regimen similar to Dr. Atkins's—without the androgen blockade—if his own urologist recommended a period of watchful waiting.

## PC-SPES

Dr. Atkins is a clinician using an empirical, broad spectrum approach that may be helpful to patients with prostate cancer but has not yet been scientifically evaluated. Dr. Sophie Chen is a biochemist with an interest in carefully studying particular Chinese herbal combinations for the treatment of specific cancers.

Dr. Chen has a long-standing interest in the development of natural products as the source of pharmacologically active therapies. In 1993, she founded International Medical Research and began to develop a combination for the treatment of prostate cancer, which she called PC-SPES. PC-SPES includes 8 different herbs, among them glycyrrhiza (licorice), the ganoderma or Reishi mushroom, 5 other TCM herbs, and 1 American herb, saw palmetto (serenoa repens).

Saw palmetto is regarded as an effective treatment for benign prostate hypertrophy (BPH) and is presently being tested for its efficacy in clinical trials. Saw palmetto inhibits the metabolism of testosterone and has a powerful anti-inflammatory and antiedema action. Dr. Chen has made the important observation that this herb's action may also prevent the promotion and proliferation of cancer cells.

In her presentation, Dr. Chen began with some epidemiological data. Men in Asian countries, she told us, have an equally high incidence of prostate cancer as North American men, but their cancer cells stay very small and are far less likely to grow and metastasize. Dr. Chen and others theorize that this is because of a diet high in soy and vegetables. Just as these dietary patterns are important to prevention, so, she believes, they might contribute to stopping the growth and spread of prostate cancer after it has been diagnosed.

Dr. Chen went on to report on her laboratory and animal testing, as well as a recent study on men with prostate cancer. In laboratory testing, PC-SPES shows action on a variety of different biological pathways. It encourages DNA repair, acts as an immune enhancer, suppresses androgen receptors, inactivates the PSA gene, and induces apoptosis. Both hormone dependent and hormone independent cancer cell lines decreased in numbers when the herbal mixture was added. This multifaceted activity, which was found against multiple cancer cell lines in the laboratory and in animal testing as well, inhibits both the progression of malignancy as well as cell growth.

Dr. Chen also reported on a clinical study of 34 prostate cancer patients with all stages of disease. Of those given PC-SPES, 90 percent had a decrease in PSA in three months and 70 percent had a drop of more than 50 percent; only 1 patient did not respond at all. Other studies are being done.

Dr. Chen reminded us that this kind of nontoxic treatment is very important, but that other factors, including dietary modification, meditation, and other relaxation techniques, are necessary for optimal care of patients. The idea, she says, is to treat the patient in ways that are both less invasive and supportive of each individual's capacity for self-healing.

In his comments, Dr. Fair called PC-SPES one of "the most exciting" new treatments for prostate cancer. Chemotherapy, he reminded us, must be potent by itself and often has quite damaging side effects. By contrast, this herbal mixture works in a synergistic and nontoxic way, with each of the herbs seemingly enhancing the effectiveness of all the others. When Dr. Chen's work was challenged in an article in the *New England Journal of Medicine,* which pointed out the anti-androgen effects of PC-SPES, Dr. Fair reminded us that the PC-SPES's antiandrogen effect is only one of many; most important, he added, cells and tumors that were not sensitive to an-

drogens were also stopped from growing and spreading (in laboratory and human studies done at the University of California, San
Francisco).

### Aged Garlic

Dr. Richard Rivlin, a professor of medicine at Cornell Medical
School and New York Hospital, spoke at the CCC about the use of
garlic as a complementary treatment for prostate cancer and more
generally about guidelines for investigating natural therapies.

Dr. Rivlin, like Dr. Chen, framed his discussion by citing epidemiological evidence. A number of studies, he explained, have shown
that the prevalence of prostate cancer is significantly lower in individuals who consume garlic and that those who consume more (and
those who consume garlic supplements as well) have even lower
rates. These studies have been done in England, China, Italy, and the
United States. He also pointed out that his research, like Dr. Chen's,
demonstrated that every stage of cancer cell growth and development could be thought of as an opportunity for intervention.

The epidemiological data and this perspective on intervention
have led scientists, including Dr. Rivlin, to a more detailed investigation of garlic. In several studies in cell cultures and animals, they
have found that water-soluble garlic extract acts against cancer in a
variety of ways. It inhibits DNA damage; inhibits prostate cancer
cell growth; reduces tumor markers, including PSA and acid phos-
phatase; accelerates the excretion of the male hormone testosterone;
and inhibits the growth of new blood vessels.

Dr. Rivlin, a distinguished mainstream scientist with impeccable
credentials, believes that the data on garlic, and other natural products, eventually will establish new guidelines for nutrition and treatment. He concluded by reminding us of the time-tested power of
phytonutrients. Old wives' remedies that have been scorned by the
medical establishment have provided the basis for many modern
pharmaceuticals, from foxglove (digitalis) to treat heart failure, to
periwinkle (vincristine and vinblastine) to treat a variety of cancers.

Garlic (and the phytonutrients we discuss in Chapter 8) may well prove to be of equal or greater importance.

## Summing Up . . .

Sitting at CCC I, Steve felt his mind was opening. He respected scientific authority and he was beginning to see that science—and scientifically based medical treatment—might be more subtle, more complex, and even more natural than he had imagined. As we sat with him and Grace after the conference we began to sketch out what we had learned, from these panels and others, and to work out some guidelines with and for him, and for others with prostate cancer.

Because prostate cancer is so common and is not always symptomatic or lethal, complete reliance on early screening as a guide for treatment is not established. Treatment decisions should not be made in haste. Any man needs information on the stage of his disease and all the treatment options, but decisions about treatment should not be made in haste. We have heard reports, good and bad, after surgery, but almost every patient complains about presurgical ignorance. In early stage disease, for some men, waiting and carefully monitoring the prostate is appropriate.

When surgery (radical prostatectomy) is indicated, according to studies done by the Institute of Medicine, the skill of the surgeon directly influences outcome. The side effects of radiation as well as surgery (impotence, incontinence, and rectal problems) can seriously affect quality of life and are sometimes irreversible. Better results with fewer complications are reported in designated cancer centers and some university hospitals. Patients need truthful and timely information, including information on the experience and record of the surgeon and radiation oncologist.

Prostate cancer seems to be almost universal, but dietary and lifestyle factors in some cultures help prevent progression. Many studies (an RCT is also in progress) suggest that a diet low in fat, high in fresh fruits and vegetables, and including soy products, green tea, garlic, and the essential fatty acids found in fish oil and flaxseed provides general protection for the prostate.

Other supplements, recommended by clinicians, include selenium, vitamin E, the B vitamins, calcium, and magnesium.

Other complementary treatments are available, including, most particularly PC-SPES, which appears to hold much promise. Other approaches, including many of those offered by Dr. Atkins, may have some value, but have not yet been adequately demonstrated.

Lifestyle changes discussed earlier, including exercise, meditation, and group support, should be included in every treatment plan.

## Breast Cancer

Grace came to the Comprehensive Cancer Care conference in good spirits. Months before, she had had a breast-conserving lumpectomy with a sentinel lymph node biopsy. When no lymph node involvement was detected, her prognosis and her mood improved. She was satisfied with her conservative surgical treatment and hopeful about her future. Her fatigue from the radiation had been distressing but manageable. She was involved in her exercise program again. Now, she was looking for ways to reduce the risk of recurrence. The chance to address her concerns to the medical experts at the CCC and to exchange stories and information with other women was exactly what she wanted and needed. She was looking for things she could do.

Grace pointed out the difficulties Steve had faced; many of them, she felt, were gender-related. Talking about intimate details, especially his reproductive system, was not easy for Steve. Prostate cancer had made him even less open. He also had had a fairly rigid belief in the power of science and technology. His experience was entirely focused on identifying the problem, finding the solution, and eliminating the problem. This single-minded pursuit of defined goals made him a successful businessman. But it had left him feeling powerless in his new reality as a cancer patient.

Grace, by contrast, had learned the value of change in her business and family life. She felt that her cancer was encouraging her to be more connected to others who had similar diagnoses. The fact that breast cancer, and information on its treatment, has had a high public profile, and that celebrities were talking about their experiences, seemed to her to make more people aware of and sensitive to her problems.

Today, most breast cancers in the United States are found during self-examination (as Sarah did) or by accident, by the patient. Depending on individual risk factors, yearly mammograms are recommended for all women over the age of 50, and all sexually active women should receive gynecological examinations regularly, including breast examinations. Eighty percent of all breast cancer is now detected in the early stages, when it is confined to the breast and nearby lymph nodes. Large-scale studies of breast cancer have established that early detection and prompt treatment offer women the best chance for cure.

Understanding the disease and one's personal risk is complicated by reports of conflicting studies on risk factors, disputed screening guidelines, and new treatments. As Grace soon discovered, regular mammograms and examinations offer no definite protection against the development of cancer. What her continuous attention did provide was earlier diagnosis and better options.

The confusion about what "risk" means creates many problems, one of which is that most women overestimate their risk of breast cancer and underrate their risk of heart disease, which is the number one cause of death among women. This may mean women do not take steps to protect their hearts and are, at the same time, unrealistically fatalistic about breast cancer.

The strongest risk factors for breast cancer are

- Age 50 or older.
- Close family members with breast cancer (mother, sister, aunt, grandmother).
- A prior history of breast cancer.
- Atypical cells on previous biopsy.

Other factors include being childless or older than age 30 at time of first giving birth; early age at onset of menstruation, and late menopause; and obesity. Prolonged hormone replacement therapy is a risk factor. Some studies indicate strong connections between diet and exercise patterns and all cancers, particularly breast cancer. Others, including some presented at the CCCs by public health advocate Devra Davis, Ph.D., suggest the deleterious effect of environmental influences, including herbicides, pesticides, and the hormones and antibiotics that are given to livestock. These toxic substances are concentrated in breast tissue, bind to estrogen receptors, and can cause damage to cells and their DNA.

Every woman should evaluate what the risks and contributing influences are in her own life. This information can lead to sensible changes that reduce risk, to paying careful attention to screening guidelines if the risk can be assessed as high, and even to taking action on environmental issues.

### What Grace Learned at the CCC

Grace helped us develop a list of some of the treatments she had found helpful and new information she gathered at the CCC. The most important, we agreed, were the self-care strategies covered in the earlier chapters of this book, including the mind-body approaches, relaxation, imagery, and exercise—and her meetings with Steve and Father Brennan.

Grace had also found her support group especially helpful. Meeting with other women who had breast cancer gave her a safe place to talk about her fears and concerns. The group was also a great resource center, a place to discuss diet, supplements, the side effects of treatments, difficulties with doctors, the fears of spouses, and the specter of death. It was also, she later reported, a wonderfully appreciative group with which to share the information she brought back from the CCC.

Because so many studies on CAM therapies—and on conventional therapies as well—have been done on women who are at risk for or have breast cancer, Grace was able to bring back information that was immediately applicable to her situation. Much of this information is presented in our chapters on diet and nutrition and phytonutrients. Following are some of the highlights and their relevance to women with breast cancer:

- Fresh vegetables and fruits provide a wide variety of substances that stimulate and support the immune system, including antioxidants and isoflavones. They are also rich in the fiber that facilitates estrogen excretion and decreases the burden of environmental toxins.
- Flavinoids present in citrus fruit act as antioxidants and reduce damage to normal breast cells.
- Although the studies are not definitive or unanimous, it appears that a diet low in animal fat may help prevent recurrences, as well as onset, of breast cancer.
- Omega-3 fatty acids specifically inhibit the growth of mammary cancer cells in test animals.
- Green tea consumption by women with breast cancer has resulted in fewer positive lymph nodes, increased disease-free survival, and decreased recurrence rates. These effects are probably due to several distinct modes of action: Green tea inhibits cancer growth by blocking growth factors or tumor promoters, by strengthening the cell walls of capillaries, and by inhibiting tumor invasion and the development of new circulation.
- Coenzyme Q10, which was used in the Danish study on women with breast cancer that we cite in Chapter 8, may significantly prolong survival in women with recurrences and metastases.
- Melatonin has a significant antiestrogen effect that is different from but complementary to that of tamoxifen. It may well, as we suggest in Chapter 8, have an important use, with and without Tamoxifen. It should be used under medical supervision.

Grace is planning to make significant changes in her diet, markedly increasing her intake of fresh fruit and vegetables and particularly citrus. She'll adapt the supplement plan in the nutrition chapter, add several cups of green tea daily, and begin to take 300 mg of Coenzyme Q10 each day.

## To Eat Soy or Not to Eat Soy

Grace was particularly interested in the presentations on soy and breast cancer. She noted that epidemiological studies show that Asian women who include soy products as a significant part of their diet regularly have lower rates of breast cancer, and that rates of colon cancer for women and men were as much as 50 percent lower in Asian populations that frequently consumed miso soup (made from fermented soybeans). Animal studies, she learned, support these findings: One study found that rats fed miso exhibited reduced incidence and decreased tumor growth in mammary adenocarcinomas.

The volume of research into soybeans and findings of its anti-carcinogenic activity have increased exponentially in recent years. Biochemical research identifies at least two kinds of active ingredients in soybeans and in such soy products as tofu and soy milk. First, there are a number of natural protease inhibitors, agents that protect normal cells from disruption and improve the functioning of immune cells. Second, and probably most important, the isoflavones that are present in soy and a variety of legumes have a number of anti-cancer activities.

The data on genistein, an isoflavone prominent in soy, show that:

- It is, itself, a "weak" estrogen that has an affinity for estrogen receptors and can therefore decrease the ability of the woman's own estrogen to bind to breast tissue and stimulate the growth of cancer.
- It induces apoptosis in cancer cells.
- It inhibits angiogenesis.
- It induces differentiation in cancer cells.

A number of researchers cite evidence on the positive effect of soy's weak phytoestrogens on preventing breast cancer and assume that the same effect will continue after a woman has breast cancer. They recommend increasing soy intake considerably. The use of soy products by women who have breast cancer is, however, very controversial. At the CCC, Dr. Charles Simone, an oncologist who is expert in complementary nutritional therapies, expressed the opinion that reducing total estrogen in the body has primary importance and that women with breast cancer should avoid all exogenous estrogens, including soy.

We believe it is also important to add that postmenopausal women without breast cancer who want to protect against both heart disease and cancer should as a rule use soy and soy products rather than tablets of pure extracted genistein and/or daidzein (another active isoflavone). We know the positive effects of soy as a whole food. We don't yet know what the risks and benefits are of long-term use of very high doses of one or more of its active weakly estrogenic components.

The decision about whether and how much soy to take was not easy for Grace. Her cancer was estrogen-positive, but she was also postmenopausal and worried about the effect of low estrogen levels on her heart and bones. The nutritionist she and Steve consulted after they returned home suggested a middle course between eliminating and adding to her soy intake: She advised Grace to continue her moderate intake of soy and soy products—about 35 grams a day—and increase the amount of fiber to shorten the time any estrogen would remain in her colon.

There is currently underway a long-term clinical study on the use of soy, antioxidants, reduced calories, and a high-fiber, low-fat, vegetarian diet, and green tea in women with breast cancer who have also received conventional care. Grace and her nutritionist know that until this study is completed, they won't have definitive information on the effect of nutritional strategies on recurrence of breast cancer or on the benefits or drawbacks of soy. In the meantime, they're responding as best they can based on the evidence we do have.

## Next . . .

Steve and Grace called the other day to report on their progress. Grace said that because antioxidants may stop DNA damage, and DNA damage is the object of radiation, her radiologist had suggested she stop taking antioxidant supplements during treatment. Grace did, although she knows there are many studies showing that antioxidants enhance the therapeutic effects of radiation. It just made her "too nervous" to go against his advice. Now she is back on all her supplements and her full regimen, fully in charge of her care, and feeling "great." As for Steve, his PSA is still slightly elevated, and he'll have another ultrasound (TRUS) examination soon. He sees the urologist every two months, for now, carefully monitoring his prostate.

Steve says he still wishes the cancer was out, gone, surgically removed. But after several consultations, the best thing to do seemed to be to wait and see. He likes definite answers but he knows the benefits of surgery in his case are not balanced by the risks. He's made changes in his diet that he learned about at the CCC, has begun to take PC-SPES, and is, to his great surprise, joining a support group.

Steve still thinks surgery is in his future. Merely controlling cancer still doesn't feel quite right to him. But right now he is doing more to enhance his life and worrying less about his prostate cancer and Grace's breast cancer and more about fishing. He's enjoying the long-term strategy he's developed: taking his herbs and eating the low-fat, high-fiber, high-soy diet that gave him a leaner body and may help control his prostate cancer.

Their daughter, Ellen, reported that Steve and Grace are, as she put it, joined at the hip again, finishing each other's sentences and planning a trip to Europe.

*Funny, Mom is more independent because of her cancer, and I think Dad finally recognized his dependence on her. So their relationship is more balanced. In fact, the whole thing has been about balance, in some way, for all of us. Cancer changed everything, and not all negative changes, either. Amazing.*

# 10

# Therapeutic Diets

ALTHOUGH MOST NUTRITIONAL approaches to cancer treatment are nontoxic and can be considered part of a healthy lifestyle, they have long been controversial. Until recently, diet has been regarded as possibly useful for prevention but quite dubious as a mode of cancer treatment. Many patients consider making major changes in their diet to be tough and anxiety provoking, while oncologists have been concerned that patients will forgo proven conventional therapy or somehow debilitate themselves by unbalanced and overly restrictive diets.

In recent years, however, we have found that physicians and those who advocate dietary treatments of cancer are moving toward a common ground. There is a growing agreement among scientists that nutrition may play a significant role in preventing cancer and that the food we eat can affect the growth and development of cancer at every stage.

For example, we now know that the antioxidants in fresh vegetables bind with free radicals. Uncontrolled free radicals cause damage and possible mutations in the structure of DNA. Eating a diet rich in antioxidants and taking supplements may help prevent malignant transformation. We know that more fiber in the diet increases the elimination of chemical carcinogens and cancer-promoting hormones, and that a vegetarian diet, especially one that is high in fiber and low in fat, helps patients maintain an ideal weight. Obesity, we have discovered, is a known risk factor for many cancers, including breast cancer, and calorie reduction may be as useful in inhibiting the recurrence of cancer as it is in preventing cancer itself.

Two of the therapeutic diets we discuss in this chapter, the Gerson diet and the macrobiotic diet, are well-known, and controversial, cancer treatment strategies. They are powerful therapeutic approaches and can be dangerous if not followed with common sense, self-awareness, and solid information. Physicians, patients, family, and caregivers must know what they are doing, must watch for changes, and must use these diets in conjunction with professionals who are experienced in supervising them. The third approach is more moderate, but still demanding: a complete dietary regime that has been integrated with a program of comprehensive cancer care by Dr. Keith Block.

Although there are significant differences among them all, the diets we cover here require discipline and commitment and take considerable time and effort for the assembly and preparation of required foods. This discipline and the routine devotion of time and mindful effort to food preparation may well be an intrinsic, if as yet unstudied, part of the process of healing; they are certainly aspects of traditional healing systems and of spiritual disciplines as well.

## The Gerson Diet

The German physician Max B. Gerson first used nutritional interventions in the treatment of migraine headaches, arthritis, and tuberculosis of the skin. In early twentieth-century Europe, where Dr. Gerson received his medical education, such approaches were part of standard medical practice.

Dr. Gerson's results in treating chronic diseases were reportedly successful and he became very well known in the 1920s and 1930s. He first expanded his treatment to include patients with cancer when a woman with bile duct cancer that had metastasized to the liver pleaded with him to work with her. She went on the diet Dr. Gerson prescribed and, according to reports published in journals at the time, had a remarkable recovery. Gerson continued to work with people with advanced cancer, apparently obtained good results, and published widely in European professional journals. In 1938 Gerson emigrated to the United States, and in 1939, having passed the state medical boards, he began to prescribe and adjust his nutritional model for U.S. patients.

Dr. Gerson believed that to be healed of cancer the body had to be restored with ionized minerals, natural foods, and detoxifying enemas. The essential elements in his regimen included

- Sodium restriction and potassium supplementation to restore cellular health, particularly the integrity of cell membranes. Dr. Gerson believed that cancer spreads to other tissues through weakened membranes; balancing the sodium and potassium levels in the cell would, he believed, stop cancer proliferation by strengthening cellular structure.
- Frequent regular doses of specific foods, including hourly administration of raw fruit and vegetable juices. The diet must consist of fresh, organic, pure, and carefully prepared food. These foods would, he believed, increase antioxidant levels in the blood. The increased fiber would facilitate excretion of toxins. According to Dr. Gerson's European education, poor diets provide hospitable terrain for disease.
- Fat and protein restriction to impede cancer progression. Dr. Gerson believed that metabolizing these nutrients increased oxidative damage from free radicals. He suspected that fat intake is directly related to cancer cell growth and proliferation, and he made use of the fasting and caloric restrictions that are the basis of many traditional and naturopathic practices. "Heavy foods," such as meat, were regarded as difficult to digest (or metabolize), and he believed that restricting fat and protein relieved the metabolic burden, allowing more efficient use of oxygen.
- Administration of thyroid hormone to stimulate metabolism and enzyme production. When Dr. Gerson

began his practice, clinicians regularly prescribed thyroid hormone as a general "tonic." The thyroid gland produces factors affecting growth, energy production, and other metabolic processes. Dr. Gerson believed thyroid supplements would hasten the cleansing process and improve emotional well-being.

- Frequent coffee enemas as part of detoxification and stimulation of the liver. Until the 1950s, the use of enemas and theories of "detoxification" were common, even in conventional U.S. medicine. In earlier research, coffee enemas were found to dilate the bile ducts and stimulate bile excretion and liver function.

During his lifetime, Dr. Gerson claimed dramatic results. Sometimes his claims were modest, as when, in 1949, he reported that his therapy was difficult to evaluate given the protean (constantly changing and evolving) nature of cancer, but that it seemed to relieve pain and slow cancer progression. Near the end of his life, when he rewrote *A Cancer Therapy*, he claimed that his therapy was an effective treatment for cancer, even in advanced cases. He presented 50 cases in that book, discussing patients whom he regarded as cured of serious cancers. He also claimed that his cure rate was 50 percent for advanced cancers, after mainstream treatment had failed.

A careful evaluation of the information presented as a "best case series" by Dr. Gerson in his book does not support many of his claims. Some cases lack proof of cancer diagnosis by biopsy or other methods, some offer little evidence of response to the diet, and some patients were receiving concurrent conventional therapies. On the other hand, a number of people with diagnosed disease, and even advanced cancer, did seem to live longer and suffer less than is usually seen with patients with similar disease.

Although individual patients continued to report "cures" of untreatable cancers, no controlled trial of Gerson's method was undertaken during his lifetime. More recently, however, Dr. Peter Lechner and his colleagues undertook a controlled clinical trial in Graz, Austria. As Michael Lerner points out in his fine, thoughtful book, *Choices in Healing*, this trial of Gerson's diet was flawed: Instead of randomization and careful matching, patients who chose to go on Gerson's diet were compared to those with similar diagnoses who didn't want to. Still, Dr. Lechner found that the patients who went on the Gerson regime did significantly better than those who didn't. The Gerson patients generally lived longer; had better response to conventional therapy, and fewer side effects from it; and had less pain, less weight loss, and a better quality of life.

Dr. Gerson's therapy is still practiced, primarily in Mexican clinics, and has eloquent advocates associated with the Gerson Institute in California. Over the years, Gerson's original diet has been modified. When Gerson first began using this therapy, he included 3 or 4 glasses of fresh calf's liver juice a day. The use of raw organic meat juices as part of the diet was eliminated, largely because of contamination with hormones, antibiotics, and bacteria. The number of enemas has also been decreased from as many as 8 a day to a schedule adjusted to the needs of the patient. Nutritional supplements—including vitamins and protein powders—are sometimes used. Gar Hildebrand, the director of the Gerson Institute, believes that the results the Gerson method is reporting today are similar to those Dr. Gerson achieved and that they vary significantly with the stage and type of cancer treated.

Since 1987, Mr. Hildebrand and the Gerson Institute in California have undertaken the task of reviewing and evaluating patient response to the Gerson program. At the 1998 CCC, Mr. Hildebrand presented data on recent investigations into the effectiveness of Dr. Gerson's therapy, including a retrospective review of 5-year survival rates in selected melanoma patients.

In this study, medical records of a group of patients with different stages of melanoma were carefully evaluated and their 5-year survival rates compared to the survival rates in similar studies on melanoma patients reported by the American Cancer Society. This is certainly not a randomized controlled trial, but it is a start in gathering data that may give a rough picture of the efficacy of Gerson's diet and pave the way for prospective studies. What Hildebrand and his colleagues found and presented is summarized below:

- 100 percent 5-year survival of 14 Stage I and II patients (local disease), compared to ACS reports of 82 percent 5-year survival with conventional care.
- 82 percent 5-year survival of 17 Stage III A patients (early lymph node involvement), compared to ACS reports of 39 percent 5-year survival.
- 70 percent survival of 33 Stage III A/B patients (early to late lymph metastasis), compared to ACS reports of 41 percent 5-year survival.
- 39 percent survival of 18 Stage IV A patients (distant skin and lymph metastasis), versus ACS-reported 6 percent 5-year survival rate.

Mr. Hildebrand also reported on early data that evaluated responses in non-Hodgkins lymphoma, colorectal cancer, and ovarian cancer. He found that those who followed only the Gerson program had approximately the same 5-year survival rates as patients receiving conventional treatment.

Retrospective case studies are expensive and time-consuming for a variety of reasons, and the results are open to question. The numbers are small, the treatment complicated, and the matching process between individuals and groups imperfect. Exactly how this therapy works cannot be determined from the available data. Even so, these data suggest that Dr. Gerson's diet, with coffee enemas, regularly prescribed fresh fruits and vegetables, and thyroid supplementation, showed clinical response in selected patients. This is, we believe, one kind of evidence required for further scientific evaluation, perhaps a randomized clinical trial.

## The Macrobiotic Diet

When George Oshawa introduced "macrobiotics" to Western audiences in the 1920s, it was understood as a spiritual path, a contemplative philosophy in the Zen tradition. He espoused a message of peace and healing and encouraged followers to lead a simple and integrated life, including a basic diet of brown rice, miso soup, sea vegetables, and other traditional foods. He called his teachings "macrobiotics," from the Greek *macro*, meaning great or large, and *bios*, meaning life. Oshawa believed many of the problems of the modern world, from disease to war and psychoses, stemmed from the bad choices people made in all aspects of daily life, including their diet. Oshawa taught that the key to health was proper diet.

Michio Kushi, Japanese-born like Oshawa, studied this macrobiotic program before leaving Japan for the United States in 1949. In New York, Kushi found positive changes in his health, both physically and spiritually, when he changed his own diet. He began studying and teaching macrobiotic principles and soon developed a wide following. His philosophy of simple living and a spiritual, physical, and communal discipline that respected the planet and sought inner peace gained popularity through the 1960s. There are still thousands who follow macrobiotic precepts as a way of life. In the 1980s, Kushi began placing a major emphasis on the role of macrobiotics in the prevention and treatment of cancer.

According to macrobiotic principles, the westernized diet (with overconsumption of dairy products, meat, and other fatty processed foods) results in an overaccumulation of toxins, and an imbalance of yin and yang in an individual. Kushi traces his use of the principles of yin and yang to ancient Chinese philosophical principles. His use of yin and yang is, however, rather different from the usage in traditional Chinese medicine (TCM) discussed in Chapter 6. Kushi uses the terms to describe structural differences (including listing foods as *yin* or *yang*) because he believes that westerners may be put off by the dynamic interrelationships and energetic processes described by TCM.

From Kushi's perspective, cancers can be described according to location. Cancers in the upper part of the body or in hollow organs are yin and include lymphoma, leukemia, and tumors of the breast, skin, esophagus, and upper stomach. Yang cancers are located in the lower or deeper parts of the body and include cancers of the ovaries, pancreas, and bone. Some cancers are identified as having both yin and yang forces; examples are cancers of the lung, liver, kidney, and uterus. In the macrobiotic analysis, each type of cancer requires a particular dietary approach to balance or strengthen yin and yang.

The basic macrobiotic diet includes whole grains (50 percent of the entire diet by weight); beans and bean products and sea vegetables (5–10 percent); miso, a fermented soy product used as a soup base (5–10 percent); seasonal vegetables (25–30 percent); fruits in moderation; and, sometimes, fish. All food is supposed to be organic, seasonal, and locally grown if possible. The diet is, thus, very low fat, high fiber, basically vegetarian, and emphasizes using whole, natural foods of good quality. Cereals form the basis of the diet, and fish is preferred to meat. Kushi explains that foods originating farther down the biological and evolutionary tree of life are healthier for any species.

Dr. Lawrence Kushi, the son of Michio and Aveline Kushi, is an academic and an epidemiologist. He is also a lifelong follower of macrobiotics, which he says is both a social movement and a nutritional and spiritual way of life. At the 1998 CCC, Dr. Kushi mentioned that he had never, to his knowledge, eaten red meat, not even chicken. The fact that most of his audience found this amazing shows how ubiquitous and accepted the Western diet, with its regular inclusion of meat and dairy in the meals of adults, has become.

Although a popular movement, especially among young students and academics, the macrobiotic diet was often attacked in the 1970's by Western orthodoxy. The *Journal of the American Medical Association,* for example, condemned the "Zen macrobiotic diet" as deadly, and reported "cases of scurvy, anemia, hypoproteinemia, hypocalcemia, emaciation due to starvation, and other forms of malnutrition, in addition to loss of kidney function. . . . When a diet has been shown (to cause) irreversible damage to health and ultimately led to death," the *JAMA* concluded, "it should be roundly condemned."

The perception of macrobiotics is very different today. The guidelines for the macrobiotic diet are, in fact, not terribly different from those of the American Cancer Society:

- Choose most of the foods you eat from plant sources.
- Limit your intake of high-fat foods, particularly from animal sources.

Other ACS recommendations regarding exercise and limiting alcohol are also part of the macrobiotic way, as are meditation, simple living, and membership in a larger community of like-minded people. The entire macrobiotic program is, in fact, a kind of therapeutic lifestyle.

People who follow a macrobiotic lifestyle have been the subject of research for many years. Studies have shown more favorable cardiovascular profiles, lower cholesterol levels, and the protective benefits of eating soy products (for example, a lower incidence of breast cancer). These results are similar to those we've seen in studies of other vegetarian and traditional Asian diets. One early and continuing criticism of macrobiotics has concerned the difficulty some people have in digesting brown rice. Most practitioners, including Dr. Kushi, advocate the use of pressure cooking techniques to make rice and other foods easier to digest.

At the 1998 Comprehensive Cancer Care conference, Dr. Lawrence Kushi began his discussion of macrobiotics and cancer by mentioning books written by cancer patients who found that macrobiotics extended and enhanced their lives. These anecdotal accounts popularized the idea of the healing power of macrobiotics and inspired many who already were inclined to believe in nutritional therapies and natural healing to undertake the rigors of macrobiotic eating. A number of these people who claimed to be "cured" of cancer by macrobiotics recently testified in the U.S. Congress.

Dr. Lawrence Kushi and his colleagues at the Kushi Institute received a grant in the mid-1990s from NIH's Office of Alternative Medicine to do a best case series. This study was not completed. At the Comprehensive Cancer Care conference, Dr. Kushi reviewed a few of the cases that were considered for inclusion. Several patients with advanced astrocytoma, verified independently, had reported total or partial tumor response; all were alive, years later, after following a macrobiotic diet, and all had normal activity. In one case, the attending neurosurgeon called the remission "a remarkable event." Dr. Kushi also mentioned, but didn't elaborate on, cases of malignant melanoma and pancreatic cancer. Unfortunately, the findings he reported were given without supportive data. We should, however, mention that it is common practice, in scientific research, to report early or preliminary information. The best case study was never finished.

With or without a completed best case series, the macrobiotic diet continues to be one of the most common dietary therapies for cancer. Both from the literature on health-promoting effects of a largely vegetarian diet and from research into specific nutrients such as soy products, we certainly can say that the standard macrobiotic diet is healthy for most people and that the macrobiotic practitioners' use of meditation, exercise, and community support are also known promoters of health.

The bottom line is that there are impressive anecdotal reports, some good reaons to believe the macrobiotic diet may have significant health value, and no hard evidence to verify its efficacy in the treatment of cancer. This is the challenge for Dr. Kushi and his colleagues, and for scientific research generally. Dr. Kushi and the Kushi Institute are rising to this challenge. They are establishing procedures for evaluating the progress of patients who seek advice for cancer treatment through the Institute. In addition, they are presently seeking data for a retrospective study, this time meeting the NCI best case series criteria.

## The Block Medical Center

Dr. Keith Block, who presented data on his treatment protocol at the 1999 Comprehensive Cancer Care conference, is the director of the Block Medical Center in Evanston, Illinois, medical director of The Cancer Institute at Edgewater Medical Center in Chicago, and research assistant professor of Medical Dietetics and Nutrition at the University of Illinois in Chicago.

Dr. Block developed an interest in alternative treatments soon after he entered medical school. He had a chronic illness that was un-

responsive to conventional therapy and, after trying different remedies, finally found relief by following a macrobiotic diet. He became
a physician committed to investigating the macrobiotic approach to
health.

After completing his residency training, Dr. Block began to separate himself from macrobiotics and develop his own comprehensive
treatment program. This now includes inpatient care at the Edgewater Medical Center in Chicago, as well as outpatient care at the
Block Medical Center.

Dr. Block bases all care on individualized, patient-centered programs, utilizing conventional care (including chemotherapy and radiation), mind-body interventions, therapeutic nutrition, phytomed-
icines, and physical care strategies. We chose to present his
approach (one of several discussed at the CCC and covered on the
CMBM Web site) in this chapter as a model of the developing field
of integrative medicine and of a program in which nutrition is regarded as central to comprehensive care.

The diet Dr. Block uses is both specific to each individual and part
of a series of interventions that he plans with each patient. Dr. Block
encourages patient involvement in every treatment decision. He believes this inclusion allows patients, who are dealing with a life-
threatening and debilitating disease, the ability to regain and
strengthen their sense of control and power. Every measure employed in his center is an opportunity for healing, education, self-
awareness, and action. Every meal, every medication, and every exercise serves this function and embodies this belief.

The basic diet at the Block Center is low in fat and high in fiber;
emphasizes soy products, whole grains, fruits, vegetables, and green
tea; and includes selected supplements. All the foods are certified organic and free of chemicals. Fish, and sometimes poultry, is provided for patients who require it. Throughout, Dr. Block emphasizes
the importance of choice—too many patients have reported a loss of
personal control, and this may well have a negative effect on outcome.

Dr. Block believes treatment should include practical advice on
specific dietary measures that increase energy levels, boost the im-

mune system, reduce nausea and other side effects of conventional treatment, and improve mood and the ability to concentrate. Dietary prescriptions can use fat restrictions and the addition of Omega-3 fatty acids to help control the levels of hormones that are known promoters of cancer growth.

Patients are also taught to use nontoxic botanical herbs and nutrients with specific pharmacological activities as part of their diet; for example, garlic to inhibit angiogenesis and enhance immunity, and the Indian spice, turmeric, to act as an antioxidant and prevent inflammation. This information and the direct experience of an effective response—such as using ginger tea for nausea—greatly increases patients' confidence, engages them in their own treatment, and improves their ability to recover.

With 15 years of clinical experience, Dr. Block reported that the diet has several major benefits:

- Patient involvement in dietary planning means many people feel a strong sense of control over their disease; they understand that they are doing something for themselves in their struggle with cancer.
- Conventional treatments have fewer side effects when nutritional strategies are used: Patients in his practice report reduced pain, nausea, vomiting, and skin irritations.
- Although precise studies are not complete, Dr. Block reports that some patients experience tumor response, including slower rates of growth, fewer metastases, and increased survival time.
- In very advanced cancers, quality of life is enhanced, with more activity and less pain.
- Malnutrition, often a direct cause of death in cancer, is rare among patients following the Block regimen. The emphasis on choice, and maintenance of appetite, through tasty, varied, well-seasoned foods, improves nutritional status.

## A Last Word

While the research data are inevitably slow to accumulate on systems like the Gerson diet and macrobiotics and on the efficacy of comprehensive and individualized programs like Dr. Block's, more and more patients—and the many clinicians who come to the CCC—are looking with increasing interest at nutrition as an integral part of all cancer care. You should indicate to your oncologist that you want and expect thoughtful and informed nutritional counseling. Good nutritional counseling is or should be an integral part of all good medicine.

If you want further help and information about developing a personal strategy, we've included suggestions for books and programs in Appendix A.

# 11

# Changing the Paradigm
# of Cancer Care:
# Drs. Burzynski and Gonzalez

CANCER SURVIVORS LIKE Mary Jo Siegel and Cheryl Wilkens make some scientists uncomfortable, not because science questions their survival of catastrophic cancer, but because medical science has few mechanisms to evaluate the extraordinary and improbable individual experience.

The gold standard of proof of effective therapeutic intervention—the careful, controlled, and statistically adjusted study—remains the randomized clinical trial. RCTs, by definition, are stripped of any individual narrative. They are evaluated by statistical, numerical standards. Therapeutic regimens are judged by the standards of what works in acceptably large numbers within certain parameters. The unusual, the surprising, the individual whose experience is too far outside the curve is, if not eliminated from consideration, at least out of focus.

Science and medicine, however, advance by bringing these unusual findings, these unique individuals, these anomalies, into focus. Sometimes they turn out to be artifacts, purely random findings, or even hoaxes. Sometimes they change the course of history as well as alter the perspective of science and extend the reach of medicine. The understanding that the sun, not the Earth, was at the center of "our" solar system came to Copernicus because he refused to ignore anomalous astronomical findings. The field of mind-body medicine opened up because researchers refused to dismiss as a hoax the abilities of yogis to alter their autonomic nervous systems. The treatment of cancer patients may expand and evolve as we observe and examine therapies that seem at first glance as anomalous as the extraordinary results they are reported to yield.

## Stepping Outside the Mainstream

Mary Jo Siegel was not ready to accept the choices she was given when she was diagnosed with non-Hodgkins lymphoma in 1991. She and her husband, Steve Siegel, consulted physicians at the University of Southern California, UCLA, the Stanford Medical Center, and the Dana Farber Cancer Institute in Boston. The Siegels report that they were informed by the most distinguished oncologists in the United States that no conventional treatment could cure her lymphoma. The only approach offered Mrs. Siegel was a highly experimental bone marrow transplant (BMT).

In 1992, after months of research, Mary Jo traveled to Houston, Texas, to begin treatment with Dr. Stanislaw Burzynski. Dr. Burzynski's treatment with antineoplastons—short chains of amino acids called peptides, which occur naturally in blood and urine—had reportedly obtained remissions in lymphoma patients without the debilitating and dangerous side effects of a bone marrow transplant.

Within a year, Mary Jo was in remission, a finding supported by her oncologist at UCLA, as well as by Dr. Burzynski. She remained in remission until 1995, when enlarged lymph nodes in her neck signaled a possible return of the disease. Dr. Burzynski started her on oral antineoplastons and, from 1996 until she spoke at the CCC in 1998, she had been disease free—in remission—with no clinical signs of lymphoma.

Her remission from lymphoma has made Mary Jo Siegel an advocate for Dr. Burzynski and his antineoplaston treatment and a believer in every patient's right to choose therapies whether or not the Food and Drug Administration has yet approved them. Cheryl

Wilkens's experiences with mainstream medicine have also taught her to question medical authority and look elsewhere for answers.

Ms. Wilkens had a small lump on her knee and three moles on her back removed in 1991 and was told the tissues showed no sign of malignancy. Within six months, the lump regrew, larger than before surgery. Cheryl had two more surgeries and ended up with a 15-inch scar, reduced functioning, and constant discomfort. She was also referred to an oncologist, who recommended chemotherapy and radiation. She decided to seek a second opinion.

The Mayo Clinic in Rochester, Minnesota, was her first stop. The Mayo Clinic doctors told her she had a Stage III melanoma, that it was lethal, and that the treatment (chemotherapy) offered small hope and would likely damage her kidneys, heart, and gall bladder.

At this point, Cheryl Wilkens decided to consult Dr. Nicholas Gonzalez in New York City. For three years, she followed his comprehensive regimen of profound dietary changes, cleansing techniques, and large quantities of pancreatic enzymes and other supplements. She says she is now cancer free and counts herself lucky. Other patients she knows, with cancers similar to hers, who chose chemotherapy and radiation, have either died or are being treated for relapse or progression of their cancer.

For Mary Jo and Cheryl and their families these treatments were indisputably successful and miraculous. For most mainstream physicians they were anecdotal reports, unreliable and undocumented. The response from the medical establishment, when it noticed, was dismissive and derogatory and, at times, quite antagonistic. Dr. Burzynski and Dr. Gonzalez have persisted, however, inviting and encouraging scientific evaluation of their therapies. The anecdotal reports have accumulated. The political activity and advocacy of patients and families (including Senator Tom Harkin, who cites his family's experience with cancer as the basis for his commitment to better, more open cancer research and health care) has escalated.

The establishment of the Office of Alternative Medicine (OAM) as part of NIH in 1992 and the development and expansion of this office into the National Center for Complementary and Alternative Medicine (NCCAM) has led to many changes. The dialogue between practitioners of what was known as "unconventional" or alternative care and the pillars of mainstream biomedical science has not only opened, but significantly enlarged and deepened. And, as time has gone on, the medical establishment has begun to cast a wary but increasingly interested eye at the methods and results of these therapies.

The presentations by Dr. Burzynski and Dr. Gonzalez at CCC I and CCC II—to commentators from the scientific establishment, to their peers, and to patients—represented an important new phase in the dialogue among cancer care clinicians and researchers, and is a crucial example of the way new and challenging therapies, and their anomalous findings, can be evaluated.

Both men are now treating patients in clinical trials designed and evaluated in collaboration with government scientific establishments, including the Food and Drug Administration and the National Cancer Institute.

## Dr. Burzynski's Antineoplastons

Dr. Stanislaw Burzynski has a clinical practice in Houston, Texas, where he also produces the "antineoplastons" he uses in his cancer treatment. His story illustrates the conflict between a researcher-clinician who discovers, develops, and prescribes a new and anomalous therapeutic agent and the mainstream cancer establishment. He has had fervent advocates and a high profile in conventional and alternative medical journals and in the general media. And he has faced extensive legal challenges, on both the federal level and in the state of Texas.

It is important to remember that most medical research in this country is sponsored by various federal agencies, from the National Institutes of Health to the Department of Defense. Pharmaceutical research is usually financed and directed by private industry and monitored by the FDA. These taxpayer-subsidized efforts are based on the understanding that the public, represented by government agencies and mandated by Congress, has an overriding interest in public health, including issues affecting individual treatment of disease. At the same time, the medical technology and pharmaceutical industries and other private sector businesses involved in health care have become huge forces in our economy. These two entities—government and private industry—are establishments with considerable power to influence all phases of health care, from basic research on the smallest molecules in a cell to how wheelchairs are designed and the control of licensing standards for medical professionals.

Individual patients and innovative practitioners have sometimes been victims as well as beneficiaries of this system. Anyone who has a chronic disease like cancer or an unconventional approach to offer soon learns about the power of economic establishments and the value of political clout. In our system, disease has an economic and political rating as well as a medical definition. For example, women had to form organizations, take to the streets, and rally both doctors and legislators to encourage new research and better treatment for breast cancer. And the power of organizations like Alcoholics Anonymous changed our cultural understanding of alcoholism from a sinful weakness to a condition worthy of understanding and amenable to appropriate therapeutic interventions. These kinds of changes take time, effort, organizing, and patience.

As an eager, precocious young student, Dr. Burzynski seemed an unlikely candidate to be at the center of controversy and this kind of social as well as scientific change. While a student in Poland, he had discovered the peptides that include what he later called "antineoplastons." At first, this was part of his basic research into the role of certain peptides in various human illnesses. In 1970, he emigrated to the United States and was invited to join the department of pharmacology at Baylor College of Medicine in Houston, Texas. By 1974, he had identified 119 peptide fractions in human urine and was beginning to investigate therapeutic possibilities.

Everything we have read and heard about Dr. Burzynski suggests that he has been, and remains, committed to open scientific investigation of his work. However, he does insist on maintaining what he regards as necessary standards and control of the antineoplastons he has been developing and prescribing. His battles with the FDA and others are less conflicts between the forces of good and evil than stories of contacts between two stubborn adversaries, neither of which recognizes the power and authority of the other. Dr. Burzynski wants to control his discovery, receive appropriate drug status, and make it available to clinicians and patients. He doesn't emphasize his financial interest but doesn't hide it either. He assumes patents and proprietary rights are part of a free market system.

On the other hand, the FDA and other government agencies are legally charged with a protective and regulatory role. And, historically, alternative therapies that may involve large sums of money are regarded with great suspicion. The FDA has developed a careful system to protect consumers and evaluate therapeutic agents. For a drug—any substance used specifically to treat disease—to reach the market, FDA approval is absolutely required.

The legal position of state and federal agencies was that Dr. Burzynski violated various laws governing FDA approval, professional standards, and interstate commerce. Dr. Burzynski and his supporters defended his professional conduct, pointing out that he consistently sought legal sanction and approval for the use of antineoplastons. The Burzynski Institute had applied for Investigative New Drug (IND) status and attempted to establish both Phase I and Phase II trials according to FDA rules.

The decades-long struggle between Dr. Burzynski and those critical of both his conduct and the efficacy of antineoplastons in cancer treatment makes an interesting and disturbing history. In the end, Dr. Burzynski was acquitted of the charges against him and the Burzynski Institute is currently conducting 72 FDA-approved clinical trials of antineoplastons for various types of cancer.

The main focus of the studies that Dr. Burzynski has undertaken is the treatment of primary malignant brain tumors, including the brain stem glioma and mixed gliomas. This focus was shaped in part by an earlier review of 40 case histories of patients with malignant primary brain tumors treated with antineoplastons by Dr. Burzynski between 1994 and 1997.

This form of review by an outside expert is, as we have said, a "best case series" report and is used by the National Cancer Institute to evaluate promising new therapies. Many conventional drugs are approved for Phase II or Phase III trials by this standard. This method does not establish how a treatment works (although researchers usually have plausible theories) but can document the clinical response, rate of response, and degree of toxicity.

The independent reviewer of Dr. Burzynski's best case series found that antineoplastons had an "impressive" 33 percent response rate, with a complete remission rate of 15 percent. Each case evaluated included precise diagnostic information on the patient who entered the treatment. These were people with particularly lethal brain cancers (with an average predicted survival time measured in months). Most had exhausted conventional treatment modalities. The rates of tumor response reported were not only "impressive," they were amazing. With these data in hand, the FDA began to work with the Burzynski Institute on designing further clinical trials.

At the 1998 CCC, Dr. Burzynski summarized his work and reported on new studies. Dr. Burzynski discussed one particular protocol suggested by the FDA in which patients outside other clinical trials were grouped together to continue treatment. In this study, 43 patients with primary malignant brain tumors were enrolled. This is a retrospective study, using patients who were already being treated with antineoplastons. The protocol is similar to an ongoing best case series. In this trial, Dr. Burzynski reported that 44.5 percent of the patients had complete and partial responses, 33.3 percent had stable disease, and 22.2 percent had progression of their cancer. Usually, patients with similar diagnoses (including glioblastoma multiform, anaplastic glioma, and high-grade astrocytoma) have a life expectancy of 6 to 9 months. These patients have survived from 2 to 12 years, as reported by Dr. Burzynski and verified by independent evaluators.

Dr. Burzynski also reported on some preliminary data in his 71 other FDA-monitored studies. The reason there are 72 different trials is that all patients at the Burzynski Institute are enrolled in clinical trials under FDA rules for INDs. Because of the long conflict between government entities, patient advocates, and the doctor, this represents a considerable compromise and a tedious process (including a massive volume of paperwork) for all involved. In any case, the data presented seemed to show that antineoplastons have a considerable, powerful, therapeutic effect in the treatment of some cancers and that further studies should be encouraged.

Dr. Burzynski, at the CCC and in other forums, has said that he believes antineoplastons, which are often significantly decreased in cancer patients, are part of a biological defense system in the body that is separate from the immune system. He believes they act on the genes, turning off signals from oncogenes and turning on tumor suppressor genes. In particular, he believes that antineoplastons inhibit the *ras* oncogene and stimulate the p53 tumor suppression gene. He may be correct. Certainly, the state of our knowledge about how all these exchanges and messages and protections operate in the body is not complete. One can easily imagine another layer of action, even another biochemical language, that contributes to—and inhibits—the complicated process of cancer initiation, promotion, and progression.

However, Dr. Burzynski presented no data to support this theory on the mechanism of action of antineoplastons. And Dr. Li-Chuan Chen, who was commissioned by NIH to evaluate the science and action of antineoplastons, was also not able to substantiate this mode of action, although he did find evidence of in vitro anti-cancer activity, cell differentiation induction, and in vivo cancer effect of antineoplastons in other studies done in China and Japan as well as in Dr. Burzynski's work.

At the 1998 CCC Dr. Arnold Eggers, a commentator who is an associate professor of neurology at SUNY Health Science Center in Brooklyn, also expressed some doubt about this mechanism of action. He pointed out that the *ras* oncogene is not implicated in glioblastoma and that p53 is seldom involved either. This certainly raises questions about Dr. Burzynski's explanation of the mechanism of action. Nevertheless, Dr. Eggers also said that the treatment data for glioblastoma with antineoplastons are "outstanding. This is," he went on, "a breakthrough in treatment for glioblastoma."

Dr. Robert Burdick, a medical oncologist who is clinical instructor at the University of Washington School of Medicine, reviewed 17 charts—a best case series of brain cancer patients—selected by Dr.

Burzynski. Dr. Burdick verified that about 15 percent had a complete response, 20 percent had partial response, 35 percent had stable disease, and 35 percent were failures. Although these findings are not as remarkable as some of Dr. Burzynski's other series, they again establish antineoplastons as having a future in the treatment of brain cancer.

Dr. Burdick did, however, raise questions about the toxicity of antineoplastons. The patients whose charts were carefully reviewed did not have any life-threatening toxicity, but three patients he followed in Seattle had severe fatigue, fever, and weakness, comparable to the side effects from conventional treatment. He also mentioned that the treatment is very expensive and must be covered by individual patients if insurance coverage is denied. (More recently, new legislation in some states has required that all experimental treatments mandated by government agencies must be accepted as insurance-covered forms of intervention.)

Two other speakers, Dr. Robert Newman (University of Texas, MD Anderson Cancer Center) and Dr. Dieter Schellinger (Georgetown, Neurology) gave their evaluations of Dr. Burzynski's data. On the basis of a magnetic resonance imaging series of 39 patients, Dr. Schellinger was able to verify both the diagnosis and the clinical results as reported by Dr. Burzynski and his associates and as evaluated by Dr. Burdick.

Dr. Newman said that, as a pharmacologist, he sees two research problems with antineoplastons. One is that this is not a single drug, but a compound. This complicates questions of both mechanism of action and the problem of selecting a specific target population who might benefit from the therapy. Second, Dr. Newman, like Dr. Burdick, has seen patients with substantial toxicity from antineoplastons, which raises questions of delivery and method, as well as dosage. He does not argue with the reported tumor response; he simply says more research in the clinic and laboratory, including independent confirmation of the antineoplastons' activity and of possible toxicity, is necessary.

This presentation and discussion about antineoplastons is exactly the kind of informed critical dialogue the CCC wants to promote, the kind of information that all patients and clinicians need to have. A treatment formerly dismissed as "alternative" at best, and fraudulent quackery at worst, is getting the careful scientific evaluation it deserves. This is an important advance in our medical and societal willingness to honestly and fairly evaluate new and anomalous cures and therapies—and a potential breakthrough discovery for cancer care.

## Testing the Limits of Cancer Care: Dr. Nicholas Gonzalez

Pancreatic cancer, which each year claims 29,000 American lives, is one of the most deadly cancers and one of the most difficult to treat. Most patients survive an average of 4 months after diagnosis. Localized pancreatic cancer, which is found in fewer than 20 percent of cases, is the most treatable; yet even with the complete surgical removal of tumors, the 5-year survival rate is only 20 percent. For patients with more advanced cancer, the overall survival rate is less than 1 percent at five years, with most patients dying within 1 year. Most pancreatic cancers are diagnosed at an advanced stage.

Treatment protocols uniformly focus on the relief of symptoms. Most pancreatic cancer patients are considered appropriate candidates for clinical trials of new treatment because the response to already available chemotherapy, radiation therapy, and surgery is so poor.

Tamara contemplated these grim possibilities and withdrew into grief and confusion. *Every day is a roller coaster ride, with fewer sensations up, and deeper, deeper plunges down. Of course I know I'm dying. I just find it hard to accept that nothing, really nothing, can be done.*

Tamara is a "woman of a certain age," surrounded by a large family, an extended group of friends, and an engaging professional life. Her recent bouts with a series of seemingly unrelated illnesses were a puzzle to everyone, including her family doctor. For several months, she suffered from extended flulike symptoms (including fever, headache, vomiting, and fatigue) and a mysterious episode of phlebitis, an inflammation of the veins in her leg. She became thin and exhausted. A woman who had always enjoyed robust health and a good life was suddenly eroded and diminished. *I began to feel like a whiny hypochondriac—all complaints, no joy. No one said so, but my family and my coworkers and even the bloody doctor began to avoid me. I knew I was sick—I could barely make it through the day. So—here's a joke—when the doctor finally ran some tests and the scan verified pancreatic cancer, I was almost relieved. Like that old tombstone joke—you know, the inscription reads "I told you I was sick." Yeah, I was sick. Dying, they say.*

Tamara cut off everyone, retreating to her bedroom, shades down, silent and still. The series of doctors she consulted were aghast that they had missed the diagnosis. It seemed to her, now, that they wanted some kind of reassurance from her. The one who had found the tumor had nothing helpful to tell her, no useful treatment. A few weeks, perhaps a few months of life was all he could see for her. Tamara wanted them all gone.

Everyone around Tamara, her friends and medical professionals—and ourselves as well—were also feeling helpless. What could any of us offer this woman who so warmly welcomed many, providing all her considerable and generous gifts of friendship, caring, and intelligence? Chinese herbs and acupuncture might ease her symptoms and slightly delay her death, massage might soothe and relax her—and we suggested them. But we realized soon that most of what we had to offer was our presence. We would be with her in the most loving way possible, helping her to go through this passage, giving and receiving as best we were able.

But we had one more idea. We had met Dr. Nicholas J. Gonzalez and attended several of his presentations at the 1998 and 1999 CCCs. We reread his findings and spoke with a few patients who were using his alternative treatment protocol for cancer. And we knew that a new clinical study specifically of his treatment for pancreatic cancer, sponsored by Columbia University and funded by the National Cancer Institute, was beginning. This Phase III trial sought to enroll 90 patients, randomized into two groups. One-half would receive standard chemotherapy and the other would follow Dr. Gonzalez's regimen.

Dr. Gonzalez had conducted a pilot study from 1994 to 1996. Eleven patients with pancreatic adenocarcinoma—8 of whom had Stage IV disease—did far better on his clinical comparison regimen than those treated with standard chemotherapy. Here are the results:

- 9 of the 11 lived one full year,
- 5 of those made it two full years,
- 4 made it to three, and
- 2 are still alive and apparently disease-free today.

By comparison, in a recent study of standard chemotherapy used in 126 patients, not one patient lived longer than 19 months. Following the presentation of his study at CCC I and prior to its publication in *Nutrition and Cancer*, the NCI had funded the clinical trial, the first study of a comprehensive alternative approach to cancer treatment ever supported by this federal agency.

### Dr. Gonzalez's Therapy

Dr. Gonzalez has been developing his protocol for almost 20 years. His original ambition as a physician, he says, did not include clinical work. He aimed to be a mainstream, Ivy League–educated, biomedical researcher, specializing in immunology, and eventually become head of a major cancer center. His ambitious career design began to change somewhat as he pursued research both in medical school and during an immunology fellowship with Dr. Robert Good, who had been director of the Memorial-Sloan Kettering Cancer Hospital in New York.

In this research, Dr. Gonzalez studied the work of Dr. William Donald Kelley, a Texas dentist who believed that cancer was at least in part caused by the body's inability to metabolize proteins. Dr. Kelley began to use large doses of pancreatic enzymes to improve the process and added individually tailored dietary plans and detoxification with coffee enemas to his cancer therapy.

In studying Dr. Kelley's theories and practices, Dr. Gonzalez came across the early twentieth-century research of Dr. John Beard, a Scottish embryologist. Dr. Beard had observed that the placenta of mammals stops growing when the fetal pancreas begins secreting pancreatic enzymes. Something in the enzymes, he theorized, brings death to the otherwise "immortal" placental cells.

Dr. Beard theorized that pancreatic enzymes might have a similar effect on "immortal" cancer cells. He began to inject the pancreatic enzyme trypsin into tumors in mice and obtained striking remissions. Before Dr. Beard's death in 1923, he documented several cases of "terminal" cancer patients treated with pancreatic enzymes. The published findings showed tumor regression and, in some cases, complete tumor remission. But medical practice, then as now, focused on the use of surgery, chemotherapy, and radiation. Few were interested in a treatment based on an unproven theory, even if the treatment seemed to work.

During his fellowship in immunology, Dr. Gonzalez pored over Beard's work and did a retrospective review of cases of 1,306 patients who had been treated with pancreatic enzymes, combined with dietary prescriptions, by Dr. Kelley. The results of his research, which eventually led to a monograph on Dr. Kelley's work, have not been published. But what Dr. Gonzalez discovered has occupied his considerable skills and intelligence in his private practice in New York. He bases his cancer treatment protocol on these decades of research.

The regimen developed by Dr. Gonzalez and now in Phase III trials (RCT) involves three interlocking strategies and enormous commitment by the patient. The Gonzalez therapy, like his mentor Kelley's, uses diet, oral supplements, and detoxification routines, including coffee enemas.

There are, according to Dr. Gonzalez, some 10 different psychophysiological types. Each presents a different picture of autonomic nervous system functioning and a different kind of acid-base balance. Sympathetic nervous system dominants have inefficient parasympathetic nervous systems and do better with plant-based diets, whereas parasympathetic dominants do better on meat-based diets. "Hard," or solid, tumors generally arise in severely compromised sympathetic dominants, while "soft" tumors (lymphomas and leukemias) are more prevalent in parasympathetic dominants. Dr. Gonzalez uses foods—special dietary regimes—to achieve both acid-base balance and appropriate equilibrium between the sympathetic and parasympathetic branches of the autonomic nervous system. Sympathetic diets are mostly vegetarian, whereas those for parasympathetic dominants include considerable meat. All foods prescribed are to be whole and organic.

The second component of Dr. Gonzalez's treatment includes the use of individually designed regimens of vitamins and minerals and concentrates of organs and glands as well as pancreatic enzymes. The pancreatic enzymes are given by mouth, every few hours, around the clock. Some patients take up to 150 pills a day for many months.

The third component of treatment—and the one that has provoked the most derision among critics and consternation among patients—is the regular use of coffee enemas. This procedure, identical to the one used in the Gerson diet, was, Dr. Gonzalez points out, a treatment listed in the mainstream *Merck Manual* until the 1970s. He believes that it causes the liver to expel toxic wastes and the gall bladder to contract. It also, Dr. Gonzalez believes, improves the excretion of the breakdown products of the cancer cells that are destroyed by the enzymes. Dr. Gonzalez couples the use of enemas with instructions on avoiding toxic chemicals in the environment, as well as in food.

Although the regime is difficult and demanding as well as highly unorthodox, Dr. Gonzalez's results have created an extraordinary demand for his program, especially among people for whom there is no promising conventional treatment or who have not succeeded with other integrative treatments, such as people with pancreatic cancer.

Gonzalez's struggle to obtain scientific review of his cancer therapy has been noted by experts in the field of medical research, as well as longtime allies of alternative medicine. After federal funding for research into "unproven therapies" became available in 1992, his consistent collection of data on his patients, including scientific verification of diagnosis, made his practice a natural choice for investigation.

But the controversy did not stop. A recent article (January 18, 2000) in the *Washington Post* raised questions about Dr. Gonzalez. The *Post* reported that, in 1994, New York regulators ordered him to undergo retraining based on criticism of his treatment of 6 cancer patients. And in 1997, the *Post* added, a Manhattan jury found Gonzalez liable for damages of $4.8 million (later reduced to $2.3 million) in a lawsuit involving his treatment of a patient with uterine cancer.

Dr. Gonzalez believes, and has evidence to substantiate it, that the findings of the State Medical Board and the outcome of the lawsuit were shaped by prejudice against alternative therapies rather than by science. The National Cancer Institute and Columbia University are sufficiently impressed with his results to continue wholeheartedly to support the scientific examination of his treatment protocol. Dr. Karen Antman, a distinguished oncologist at Columbia University, reminded the *Post* reporter that it was science, not disputed personal history, that concerned her and was of paramount importance to patients. "It's not him, it's the treatment," that is being evaluated, Dr. Antman declared. "He is willing to have [this treatment] tested in the most rigorous way."

The NCI-sponsored Phase III trial of the regimen that Dr. Gonzalez has undertaken with Columbia has, however, run into another kind of trouble: difficulty in acquiring patients. The reason is that this is a randomized trial, and people who have lethal, pancreatic cancer and are willing to commit to the Gonzalez protocol are not ready to take the chance of being randomized to *standard* chemotherapy. They all want Gonzalez's therapy. Together, Dr. Gonzalez, Columbia University, and the NCI are working to redesign the study, perhaps as a prospective trial of a large group of people whose outcomes will be compared to the results of standard treatment.

### Tamara's Dilemma

We brought all the information we could gather on Dr. Gonzalez and his treatment to Tamara. The regimen certainly was difficult and demanding and, in some ways, strange, but it offered some hope and its focus on individualized treatment and enhancing the body's capacity for self-healing made sense to us. Still, this clearly had to be her decision. She was capable of assessing the evidence and weighing the choices herself. This treatment would require her full cooperation and commitment. It also would require substantial support from her family and friends. All we felt we could do—should do—is offer the information and our help, answer questions, and let Tamara decide.

Then there were complications. Some of Tamara's family, including her father, husband, and one of her children, were adamantly opposed to Gonzalez's regime. They felt it was too weird and would be too disruptive of whatever was left of her life, and their lives as well. Tamara seemed so weak to them, and success seemed so improbable. Her mother and oldest daughter and some friends were more enthusiastic. They believed Tamara was capable of following the regimen and were ready to provide necessary support. They were impressed with Gonzalez's data and the fact that the NCI had committed its money, time, and prestige to studying this therapy. They regarded the Gonzalez treatment as we did, as her last best hope for help.

Some of Tamara's physicians were guarded but interested in the Gonzalez therapy. The family doctor suggested that it was an experimental, unproven therapy, but that the published results were better than any known conventional treatment of pancreatic cancer. One oncologist was horrified that anyone would even consider such a regimen—*coffee enemas;* another specialist reserved judgment, offering to consult with Gonzalez and "see what this would require" of Tamara, of her doctors, and of her family.

Tamara became more withdrawn and distant as the battle about her treatment escalated. *I'm tired. I think it's partly the cancer, and partly the uncertainty and the arguments. It becomes hard to believe people have my best interests at heart when they become so adamant, so rigid, so sure they're right. Dr. Gonzalez and his staff are kind and encouraging but can guarantee nothing. The family— well, they love me, but want me to be the way I've always been. Some think this regimen is so weird and drastic I'll be changed forever. Some don't care—they just want me to try anything, everything, to live, as if my death would be their failure.*

Tamara remained undecided. She asked for, and received, help in utilizing strategies to maintain and strengthen her physical, mental, and spiritual well-being. No matter what she decided, she was definitely doing some things for herself now. Her diet, always sensible, now consisted of what she called "efficient" foods, foods that stimulated her appetite and provided, as she said, "the maximum nutrition per bite." Brightly colored vegetables, herbs and spices, broiled fish and whole grains, fresh fruit and ginger tea were favorites. Small servings, lovingly prepared, and relaxed, frequent meals seemed to provide good food for her senses as well as her body.

Her children brought pets that needed company and encouraged Tamara to take short walks; an old friend who taught yoga came to stretch with her every day. Tamara also began re-reading favorites: poets she loved, the Bible, philosophy. She was still in a reserved and quiet mood, but began to call friends and tease her family. Tamara was different, her daughter said. *She's gone some place deep inside. She is just as warm and loving, but, somehow, it's as it she's building her strength by herself, underground where we can't help her or demand her attention for ourselves.*

The choice to try or not try Dr. Gonzalez's therapy was, and still remains, Tamara's. We were torn. We felt she should have tried his approach—the evidence was convincing enough, and there were no viable alternatives—but we completely understood her hesitation.

There was little doubt about the effort and discomfort that would have been involved. There would have been drastic changes in a routine that was giving her comfort, consternation and strife in her family, and, of course, no certainty of outcome.

## A Final Word

Dr. Gonzalez's and Dr. Burzynski's work are promising. We would recommend, and have recommended, their approaches to people whose tumors have resisted all conventional therapies and in cases where conventional therapies or other approaches are likely to have limited benefits. We also suggest that people approach these and other experimental therapies being tested under NCI or FDA guidelines with appropriate caution and a clear understanding of therapeutic expectations. *And*, even in recommending them, we certainly recognize that these treatments are not for everyone, even in the most extreme circumstances.

Along with Tamara and the many others who are waiting, we look forward eagerly to the results of the research on Dr. Burzynski's and Dr. Gonzalez's protocols, research we will present and evaluate at future Comprehensive Care Conferences.

In the end, Tamara asked that we not write about her decision. She felt it would violate her privacy, that the way she decided to go was not reducible to a few concluding sentences. *Tell people that all you can do is decide to live the way that is consistent with who you are. Whether you go for broke with conventional treatment, in hopes that it may work, or go for an experimental protocol like Dr. Gonzalez's, decide to do whatever it is 100 percent, trusting yourself and your healing partners. There isn't any other advice or example any of us can provide.*

# 12

## Next Steps

### Dr. Fair's Tumor

In 1994, Dr. William Fair found himself transformed from doctor—chairman of the Urology Department at Memorial Sloan-Kettering Cancer Center—to patient, a man diagnosed with cancer of the colon. Surgeons removed the tumor and found that two lymph nodes were involved. His 5-year survival odds were 40/60. The presence of cancer in the lymph nodes suggested that there could be other sites involved, tumors too small to identify during surgery. In other words, the probability was that he had metastatic colon cancer.

Dr. Fair was aware that his colon cancer was regarded as resistant to both chemotherapy and radiation. His best hope had been the possibility of complete surgical excision of the tumor. Now, he faced a year of chemotherapy as well, hoping it would destroy any hidden cancer cells and raise his 5-year survival chances to 50 percent. Because he was a surgical oncologist, Dr. Fair never doubted or denied his diagnosis, the efficacy of conventional treatment and regular follow-up, or the prognosis. He knew, and accepted, the experts' word as truth. The knowledge and experience of a lifetime made him very realistic about his odds.

Dr. Fair says he had the finest conventional care medicine could offer. For a year after the completion of aggressive chemotherapy, he chose to believe life would go on as usual, that his cancer was gone. Then, in 1997, a routine CAT scan showed the cancer growing near his liver. His chances of survival fell, and so did his spirits. Dr. Fair knew that mainstream medicine had little to offer. His oncologists knew he knew there was no evidence to support another, more toxic and debilitating round of chemotherapy. Still, they offered this as his best option.

When Dr. Fair tries to help people understand why doctors propose treatments that offer little help to their patients he explains, with his own experience to guide him, that doctors want to help, want to do *something*. "Even if it's a one in a million shot . . . it's very difficult for a physician to say we have nothing to offer." With some irony, he suggests this does offer *hope* to the patient. Personally, he was ready to try other options and decided to avoid another round of chemotherapy.

At the first Comprehensive Cancer Care conference, and later in an interview on television and an article in the *New Yorker* magazine, Dr. Fair discussed the integrative healing program he has created for himself and the changes it has made in his cancer and his life.

Dr. Fair has spent his professional life in the hard-charging climate of one of the major cancer centers in the world. He is a urologist, a surgeon who specializes in cancers of the kidney, bladder, testicles, and prostate. Such men are generals among the front line troops in the war against cancer, routinely making instant life-and-death decisions, teaching other doctors, administering a complex medical world. This work requires a decisive, energetic, and powerful personality.

When he speaks now, it is hard to think of Dr. Fair as a surgeon. In person, he seems calm and slightly amused, intelligent and soft-spoken. He says his expectations of his program of complementary therapies were modest. He was looking, he said, for "life expansion rather than life extension."

Dr. Fair took his first steps on his program of life expansion after his wife insisted that he begin to address the psychological and spiritual dimensions of his dismal prognosis, that whether or not he believed in them, he needed to start considering some alternatives.

When he talks about that time, several years after his struggle began, Dr. Fair is both bemused and amused. "Look," he says. "When what you've been doing is not working, all this business about trying to play the tough guy has got to change." For years he had dismissed the self-care strategies we've discussed, including meditation, yoga, imagery, dietary changes, and supplements, as "New Age stuff." But as he began to go through the research on them, he was impressed.

Dr. Fair spent some time at Commonweal in California, began a regular practice of meditation and yoga, explored his psychological strengths and weaknesses, and changed his diet and many of his habits. Dr. Fair's is a completely rational treatment plan, and he can offer evidence for everything he did. In the process of reviewing the scientific literature for complementary therapies, of exploring his mind and heart, and of caring for his body, he also developed an appreciation for the vagaries of chance and the healing power of intangibles, including humor and love.

Dr. Fair contacted a leading Chinese herbalist in Shanghai, who formulated an individualized combination of herbs specifically designed to control his cancer. He read the scientific literature on psychoneuroimmunology, persevered in his meditation and yoga practice, and called us up to discuss the pros and cons of various supplements and phytonutrients.

A fellow researcher harvested cancer cells from Fair's tumor. These harvested cells were injected into laboratory animals to produce tumors in them. The researcher discovered that the herbalist's formula did indeed shrink these tumors. Other cultured cancer cells were used to develop a highly experimental, individualized cancer vaccine. Presently, Fair continues on herbs and is reserving the tumor vaccine as a last resort.

"If anyone had told me four years ago that I'd be espousing yoga and meditation I would have said 'you're crazy,'" he told the *Dateline* interviewer with a smile. On television, Dr. Fair was shown meditating in a garden, walking on a beach with his wife, and being guided through yoga postures. His wife and son speak lovingly and hopefully. We see him with patients, his arm around them, gently helping them to create their own programs of comprehensive cancer care.

As of this writing Dr. Fair's CAT scans show no sign of tumor. If he needs it, down the road, he'll try the tumor vaccine. Right now, he has already exceeded, by several years, all the oncologists' projections for his life span.

Dr. Fair's program is a model of comprehensive cancer care. The changes in his tumor status, his prognosis, and his life are exactly the kind that we would wish for everyone.

We recognize, of course, that Dr. Fair's training, his professional contacts, and his finances all opened up options that are not available to everyone. However, this kind of life expansion *should be* available to everyone. People concerned with cancer care, including those who have participated in the Comprehensive Cancer Care conferences and all of you who are reading this book must become advocates of the following: integrative programs to serve as pilot studies, research to explore their efficacy, broad programs of education and prevention to decrease the incidence of cancer, and financing to pay for these programs.

While we are all working on this transformation, we urge you to look for integrative care for yourself. You probably don't work side by side with some of the most distinguished oncologists in the world, but you can pick and choose among the most effective and thoughtful ones in your community. You may not have the resources to have an individualized tumor vaccine developed, but you can certainly explore the options for immune enhancement that we've discussed in earlier chapters. You probably can't find a twentieth-generation Shanghai herbalist to design your Chinese herbal program, but you may well be able to find a Chinese physician from Shanghai, or Beijing, or a well-trained American acupuncturist-herbalist in San Francisco or Chicago or Indianapolis. If you cannot or don't want to go to Commonweal for a week, you can find a mind-body skills group or other support group in your area.

Here in this concluding section, we want to remind you that there are things that all of you can do, healing partners you can find, new attitudes and perspectives you can adopt, knowledge you can gain, techniques you can master, and resources that you can use creatively. We remind you once more of them—of possibilities, guidelines, and maps to the territory of your care—knowing that the path you take will be uniquely yours.

## Step One: You Can Do Something

The first step in creating a program of comprehensive cancer care is realizing that you have the power to do it. This shift from passivity and stoicism, from helplessness and hopelessness, to awareness and activity, is basic to all the others. It may well take time to overcome the initial shock—the fear, vulnerability, and hurt—caused by the diagnosis. It is certainly easier for those of you, who, like Sarah and Dr. Fair, have both fighting spirit and resources. It will be harder for those like Jack, the World War II veteran, who are used to putting up with bad situations. Still, this change is possible for everyone. And everything we've read, and everyone we have worked with, tells us that this shift in perspective can make a very real difference, certainly in the quality of life, and perhaps, as Dr. Fair says, in its expansion as well.

The realization that you can do something allows you to make choices about which healing partners to pick and which ones to avoid. It gives you the freedom to interpret the data you are given, as Stephen Jay Gould did, seeing yourself among those who survive, however small the percentage, rather than among those who don't. Your sense of your own power reminds you that you can find information in this text and others, online and in person, at conferences like Comprehensive Cancer Care, and in your community.

Knowing you can do something encourages you to appreciate and make use of your own insights, to become aware of thoughts and attitudes that may inhibit or frustrate or mislead you. If you can use your awareness to guide your choices, then you do not have to deny your anger or your fear. If you can realize how alone you may feel, you can then reach out to others. If, like Dr. Fair, you can accept that you need not be limited by the limitations of conventional care, you can stop being a tough guy or a victim and look around for other possibilities.

## Step Two: Finding Healing Partners

We've discussed three kinds of healing partnerships: with family and friends, with caregivers (conventional, complementary, and alternative), and with a group specifically designed for sharing your experience and enhancing your capacity for self-care. Each partnership can enrich and deepen the others.

Americans who were raised on myths of rugged individualism, tales of solitary courage, and character-building independence may look at any chronic illness as a kind of weakness. Getting the help that's needed, and knowing that you can't or shouldn't have to deal with cancer by yourself, is most obviously difficult for men: Martin the journalist, Jack the war veteran, and Tom the litigator. But it's not easy for women either. Sarah's pride sometimes hindered her progress; it took time for her to recognize how much easier recovery would be if she talked about her fears to her husband. She had to learn to ask for what she needed. Tamara wanted to be the person she was before diagnosis, and knowing this was impossible, she withdrew into solitary despair before she could consider her options.

Often other people will reach out to you, sometimes gently, sometimes insistently. This process of reaching out not only provides support, it actually enhances the capacity of the person with cancer to take control of his or her life, to care better and more for himself or herself. Ben's staunch partisanship and determined research made it possible for Clarissa to develop and follow through on a comprehensive care plan that worked for her. Dr. Fair's wife insisted, lovingly but firmly, that he look for help in what he had previously dismissed.

Sometimes, however, others may be fearful of reaching out. They may worry about intruding or misinterpret your temporary withdrawal as a rejection. So it's important to call and ask for help, not only from professionals, but also from family and friends. We were deeply touched and appreciative of Martin's desire to have us at his side in his last months. Most people we know—from Tom's son to Tamara's family—also find it satisfying to be intimate with and generous and helpful to someone who asks. It's a way to show love and be useful. And, as we've said before, if people in the family, or close friends, withdraw, let them go. They'll come back if and when they're ready.

It is obviously crucial to find the best available health care. You have to check the credentials of conventional, complementary, and alternative professionals, and of the institutions in which they work. Remember, the decisions you make about who will care for you may occasionally mean the difference between life and death and will quite often significantly affect the quality of your life.

In the course of researching breast and prostate cancer, we were stunned by the disparity between treatment options and outcomes from hospital to hospital and physician to physician. Some surgeons who had performed prostatectomies had rates of complications— impotence and incontinence—that were 25 percent, and others did significant damage to more than 80 percent of those on whom they operated. Poor women and older women had, in general, more invasive and debilitating surgery for breast cancer than women who were younger and more affluent.

And, as we've said before, technical expertise is only one part of the equation. Physicians or acupuncturists who dismiss the hard questions you ask, or who avoid the powerful emotional issues that cancer evokes, are not full healing partners. Take the time you need to find professionals who meet your needs. Don't let yourself be unnecessarily hurried. Your tumor most likely took years to grow; except in exceptional circumstances, a few extra days spent choosing a respectful healing partner will present no problem. There are many of them out there.

If you can find someone to help guide you in creating your program of integrative care—the kind of integrative care counselors we are training, a navigator like the ones at Harlem Hospital, a guide like the ones we've listed in Appendix A—please use that person. And if you would like someone to talk to about the stress of cancer and its diagnosis, find the kind of counselor we discussed in Chapter 4: a knowledgeable psycho-oncologist or other therapist.

Third, we want to remind you of the power of support groups. The ones we recommend—like those at Commonweal and at the Center for Mind-Body Medicine—are places where you can share your experience with others, become more self-aware and self-accepting, and learn the life-enhancing techniques of self-care. As you name the dilemmas you face and find others who face ones similar to yours, you feel less isolated. As you learn to better understand and care for yourself, you overcome hopelessness and helplessness.

Remember, active participation in a support group may prolong your life. The research by Spiegel and Fawzy on metastatic breast cancer and adults with malignant melanoma is not definitive, but it is certainly highly suggestive. We suggest that you explore opportunities for support groups. If one feels good to you, you have everything to gain—and nothing to lose—by joining and participating in it.

## Step Three: Self-Awareness and Self-Care

In the past, techniques of self-awareness and self-care were often dismissed as useless and, at best, regarded as ancillary to surgery, radiation, and chemotherapy. Time enough for that, many people were told, after you've recovered from the surgery and after the chemotherapy is well underway. We believe, and, increasingly, oncologists agree, that this attitude is short-sighted.

It is precisely in those first days and weeks, when you are dealing with the shock of diagnosis, the bewilderment of making choices, and the trauma of treatment, that self-care strategies—as well as group support—are vital. If you learn techniques of deep breathing, relaxation, and imagery you can often decrease the amount of anesthesia and pain medication you need, reduce the number of complications from surgery, and abate some of the side effects of chemotherapy and radiation. Equally important, the concrete experience of having some sense of control, of being able to actively participate in your own care, may make a major contribution to the quality of your life and to treatment outcome as well.

We've been extremely impressed by the experience of the people we've described in this book and by the data presented at the Comprehensive Cancer Care conferences on the effectiveness of self-expression, relaxation, meditation, imagery, hypnosis, mind-body therapies, and physical exercise, including walking, yoga, *tai chi*, and *qi gong*. We've described some specific techniques, and in Appendixes A and B we have listed many resources to help you find further information and instruction. We are convinced that this approach and these techniques should be an integral part of everyone's cancer care.

So too should a program of mindful eating. The evidence we present in Chapter 5, and the recommendations we make about diet and supplements, are an excellent place to start. Some of the books on nutrition in Appendix A provide practical help in selecting healthy foods and in preparing meals, and the books and papers listed in the Notes and Bibliography describe much of the original research on which our recommendations are based. If, as many of the leading epidemiologists say, nutrition is a factor in causing the majority of all cancers, it certainly makes sense to use good nutrition as a significant part of your program of comprehensive cancer care.

## Step Four: Balancing Treatment Decisions

In Chapter 2, "Facts for Life," we define some of the medical terms that are used to describe the biology of cancer and its diagnosis, treatment, and prognosis. We address the concepts of risk and the ways that the benefits of treatment are described. Refer back to this discussion and those definitions as you pursue treatment options. Understanding the scientific discourse about cancer care allows you to ask more intelligent questions about all the treatment possibilities that are open to you. This is a basic form of self-care, as well as a crucial strategy for helping to ensure that you get the most effective treatment.

There is no way here to suggest specific treatment options for hundreds of different kinds of cancers in the bodies of millions of unique individuals. All we can do is offer guidelines. First of all, you should look at every therapeutic option—conventional, complementary, or alternative—in a similar way, assessing the risks and benefits of the treatment. What is the scientific evidence available for its efficacy? How does the evidence relate to my particular cancer and me? Do the benefits of the treatment outweigh the risks? Will the particular treatment interfere with another I am currently receiving or one I am considering? How will the treatment affect—for good or ill—the quality of my life?

If the tumor can be removed, surgery—except in the rarest circumstances—is an obvious first choice, but one that still carries with it, as in the case of prostate cancer, very real risks. Surgery can also be used to improve quality of life and enhance longevity even when the removal of the entire tumor is impossible. Chemotherapy and radiation can also be immensely useful, but it's important to remember that all interventions must be carefully evaluated and risks and benefits realistically balanced.

Remember Dr. Fair's cautionary tale: Oncologists, like other physicians, want to do something to help, even if sometimes the chances of success are minuscule. What may look like a reasonable option from their perspective may in some instances make as little sense to you as it did to Dr. Fair.

In general, be very sure you understand the reasons why your oncologist—or complementary or alternative practitioner—recommends a particular treatment. Feel free to ask for the research supporting any recommendations. Discuss what you've heard with your other healing partners and feel free to ask for an opinion from a second oncologist. It's your care, indeed your life, that's in question.

As we've said, the same kinds of criteria need to be applied to complementary and alternative therapies as to conventional treatment. For the self-care strategies we discuss, the benefits are or may be significant and the risks are very small. With some complementary therapies, including phytonutrients, the situation may be more complex. It's quite safe to increase your intake of green tea and garlic, but, as we've pointed out, the use of other natural substances may require guidance from professionals who are familiar with both the substances and their interactions with cancer and conventional care. For example, it seems that melatonin may be extremely useful either on its own or as a complement to radiation or chemotherapy, but it is a hormone and its use should be carefully supervised. In addition, there is some evidence that it may have deleterious effects on patients with leukemia.

We believe, as we said in Chapter 6, that Chinese medicine—in particular, acupuncture, herbal therapies, and *qi gong*—can be productively integrated into the treatment of virtually everyone with cancer. These approaches are thousands of years old; there are increasingly good studies on their mode of action; and, perhaps most important, it appears that these therapies can be used safely and effectively together with surgery, chemotherapy, and radiation to enhance both quality and length of life. The issues here are finding skilled practitioners who can tailor these treatments to you and your cancer and facilitating communication between Chinese and Western physicians.

Some of the most difficult choices are about those treatments that represent alternatives to conventional approaches. The work of Drs. Burzynski and Gonzalez, as well as the uses of MTH–68/H and the Gerson diet, that were described at CCC I and II, are all representative of this category.

The clearest case for considering these therapies is if you have a cancer for which conventional oncology has no good treatment, or if you've exhausted all of the conventional treatments. At that point, a risk-benefits analysis may encourage you to expend the time and energy, to suffer whatever discomfort and significant financial investment are required, to use a therapy that seems to offer some hope. This is the case with the vast majority of parents who bring children with untreatable brain tumors to Dr. Burzynski, and with the hundreds of people with pancreatic cancer and advanced metastatic cancer who are looking for help from Dr. Gonzalez. However, even in these instances, the choice is not easy—witness Tamara's dilemma.

The choice becomes far more difficult when the situation is ominous, if, for example the tumor is metastatic, but there are still conventional remedies available. How do you compare a conventional therapy that offers some significant hope for 5-year survival, although almost no chance of cure, against an alternative that has anecdotes of cure but for which the scientific data are slim? How do you know when to choose the conventional therapy, which may in some measure diminish your natural healing mechanisms—for example, your immune system—over an alternative therapy that appears to work by mobilizing the immune system?

You need to begin by bringing together the best possible information on both the conventional and alternative approaches and by bringing the same critical eye to the evidence on all therapies. We strongly advise you to ask someone with a good analytical as well as an open mind and a medical background to assess the evidence with you. Ideally, this person would be your oncologist, but another physician, or an integrative care counselor, could also serve in this role.

Then there are situations like Steve's. In the case of his slow-growing, small prostate cancer, there may be the luxury of time to try alternative approaches first and, if they don't work, to use surgery or radiation. Here too we greatly value the personal guidance of an oncologist committed to fair-minded scientific evaluation of all therapies and deeply sensitive to the needs of patients, or of an integrative care counselor.

In the past there has been unquestioning and hasty use and sometimes overuse of conventional therapies. This is still a problem. However, it is important not to choose alternative treatments instead of conventional therapy simply because they do less harm. It's as dangerous to react against conventional treatment with dogmatism as it is to adhere dogmatically to conventional approaches. Hippocrates said, "First: Do no harm." But he also warned that "in extreme situations, extreme remedies" may be necessary.

## Summing Up

Comprehensive cancer care is grounded in self-awareness and self-care, in an open-minded and critical assessment of all therapeutic possibilities. It should be informed by the best available information and sustained by the strongest support system: family and friends, professional caregivers, and participation in a group with other people who are dealing with serious or life-threatening illness. It includes carefully thought-through and measured choices of conventional therapies, combined with proven complementary approaches and alternatives that genuinely offer more benefits than risks.

We've written in this last chapter about steps on your path. We recognize, also, that sometimes decisions must be made simultaneously and choices continually adjusted to meet the challenge of illness. So we also find it useful to think of what we've presented as a framework or scaffold that will shape and sustain your decisions, a structure on which you can lean.

Today there are far more possibilities than we could have imagined 20 years ago as we sat with Martin. There is the opportunity now to call with confidence on the wisdom of some ancient healing traditions as well as of modern research and to use modern methods to explore these traditions and their techniques. We now have a far broader perspective on ways to care for ourselves, to enhance our lives and combat our cancer. There are developments in research and more resources and more thoughtful, open-minded, informed people to support us at every step in our healing journey.

# Appendix A
# Comprehensive
# Cancer Care Resources

## *The Center for Mind-Body Medicine*
### *James S. Gordon, M.D., Director*

THE PURPOSE OF the Center for Mind-Body Medicine is to create models of healing that will transform all parties in the healing process and make those models as available, as accessible, and as influential as possible.

The Center's mission is to create and nurture a community of healers who are committed to sharing themselves and what they are learning with people with chronic illness, particularly those living with cancer; with health professionals who want to transform themselves and their practices and institutions; and with societies that are wounded and dysfunctional.

We at the Center are working to create a more compassionate, open-minded, and effective model of health care and health education. This model combines the precision of modern science with the wisdom of ancient healing. It addresses the mental, emotional, social, and spiritual as well as the physical dimensions of health and illness. It emphasizes the uniqueness of each person and the centrality of therapeutic partnerships. It is grounded in a conviction that all of us have a great and largely untapped capacity to understand ourselves, to improve our own health and well-being, and to help one another.

The Center is at the forefront of a movement that seeks to bring this empowering approach into the heart of American medical practice and to make it the core of the education of all health care providers. The Center is particularly committed to the development of new models of care; to the education of medical students and those who teach them; to service to the poor, children, the elderly, the chronically ill, and the institutionalized; and to the inclusion of volunteers in all aspects of our work.

We are actively involved in demonstrating the universal appropriateness and cost-effectiveness of mind-body medicine and to making it a shaping force in health care in the United States and internationally. Our services are available to all regardless of ability to pay.

Our programs include a professional training program; Mind-Body Skills Groups for people with cancer and other chronic illnesses; the Comprehensive Cancer Care conference; the Nutrition Training Program; and Healing the Wounds of War: A Practical Program for Dealing with Post-War Trauma and Stress.

Information about all the Center's programs is available from the Center for Mind-Body Medicine, 5225 Connecticut Ave., NW, Suite 414, Washington, DC 20015; phone 202-966-7338, fax 202-966-2589. Detailed information about all programs is available on the Center's Web site, www.cmbm.org.

## The Comprehensive Cancer Care Conferences

The Comprehensive Cancer Care Conferences (CCCs), like this book based on them, were created to answer the questions of those who have cancer and their families and the professionals who care for them. The conferences present data on which complementary and alternative therapies work and how we know that they do. They offer detailed discussions of the best integrative programs in the world and reports on the most promising therapies. The conferences present the latest information on government policy on integrative care, legislation that may promote it, and insurance companies that are likely to support it.

At the CCC, complementary and alternative researchers, clinicians, and mainstream oncologists come together with patients and their families to learn from one another and to develop together the most effective, humane, and responsive ways of treating and preventing cancer. CCCs include plenary sessions with some of the world's leading clinicians and researchers, breakout sessions presenting the most promising therapies and authoritative critiques of them, workshops to learn about and gain practical experience in nutritional and mind-body approaches, and opportunities to meet those who are offering the best care available and to ask them questions. CCC presenters include the director and deputy director of the National Cancer Institute, scientists from the NCI, the director and staff of NIH's National Center for Complementary and Alternative Medicine, the president of the American Cancer Society, outstanding CAM clinicians and researchers, patients, and patient advocates. The CCCs include representatives from most of America's leading cancer centers.

Comprehensive Cancer Care 2000 will take place June 7–11, 2000, at the Hyatt Regency Crystal City in Arlington, Virginia. To register or to receive a registration brochure, contact 202-966-7338. Detailed information about the conference is available on the Center's Web site, www.cmbm.org.

## Comprehensive Cancer Care: Integrating Complementary and Alternative Therapies Transcripts and Summaries

Transcripts and summaries of all presentations at Comprehensive Cancer Care I and II are available free of charge on the Center's Web site. Transcripts include both the original presentations and comments made on them. Summaries of Comprehensive Cancer Care 2000 will be posted by December 2000.

Comprehensive Cancer Care IV: Integrating Complementary and Alternative Therapies will take place in September 2001.

## Mind-Body-Spirit Medicine: The Professional Training Program

Each year the Center for Mind-Body Medicine offers a week-long intensive professional training program: Mind-Body-Spirit Medicine: The Professional Training Program. Participants in this program learn and experience the power of the mind-body approach and integrate its many dimensions—physical, emotional, social, and spiritual—into their personal lives and clinical practices with individual patients and clients. This intensive program is particularly helpful in preparing graduates to lead therapeutic and educational support groups for people coping with cancer and other chronic illnesses (see "Mind-Body Skills Groups").

This program, which has over 650 graduates from around the world, has been hailed by many as the "single most rewarding and stimulating training I've ever experienced." Registration and detailed information about the program can be found on the Center's Web site, www.cmbm.org.

In the year 2000, Mind-Body-Spirit Medicine: The Professional Training Program, will be held at Hilton Head, South Carolina, from November 12–18.

A list of professional training program graduates who are available to counsel people with cancer is available by calling the Center for Mind-Body Medicine at 202-966-7338, or writing to the Center for Mind-Body Medicine, 5225 Connecticut Ave., NW, Suite 414, Washington, DC 20015.

## Mind-Body Skills Groups

For 10 years the Center for Mind-Body-Medicine has offered comprehensive and groundbreaking educational groups for people living with stress or chronic or life-threatening illness. These groups, which have a special emphasis on people with cancer, give participants the opportunity to transform the physical, mental, social, emotional, and spiritual dimensions of their lives. They teach people with cancer to maximize the natural ability of their bodies to heal themselves through a variety of mind-body techniques, including self-awareness, biofeedback, drawings, imagery, meditation, breathing techniques, self-hypnosis, and movement, which have been demonstrated to be effective for improving immunity and enhancing health and well-being.

The groups, which ordinarily meet 2 hours each week for 12 weeks, include time for participants to discuss their experience of stress and illness, as well as to share and enhance their efforts to incorporate the tools of mind-body medicine into their lives. These small groups emphasize teaching and learning approaches to self-care, sharing experiences, and building support systems.

For more information about the groups, contact the Clinical Director of the Mind-Body Skills Group Program, Nancy Harazduk, MS, LICSW, at 202-966-7338. For information about Center for Mind-Body Medicine professional training program graduates who may be offering these groups in your area, please call the Center for Mind-Body Medicine.

## RESOURCE DIRECTORY

The following section is intended to assist cancer patients and their families in finding the resources they need. There are many excellent organizations across the country that are not included in the listings below. We have tried to highlight just some of the organizations that may be helpful to contact for information and support, wherever you live and whatever type of cancer you may have. We hope these organizations can provide a starting place from which to find resources that meet your individualized needs.

### National Organizations

There are several national organizations that provide excellent basic information on cancer, its prevention, and treatment options. These organizations are also good resources to begin to find local support groups and services.

*American Cancer Society.*    The American Cancer Society (ACS) offers information about cancer, treatment options, and support services. ACS has a national office where a cancer information specialist can be reached 24 hours a day and at least one local chapter in every state. These local chapters can be an excellent source of references to local support services such as financial assistance, transportation, counseling and support groups, and rehabilitation services. Although the ACS provides limited information on alternative and complementary treatments, their other services can be very useful.

Address: National Office
1599 Clifton Rd., NE
Atlanta, GA 30329
Phone: 1-800-ACS-2345 (1-800-227-2345)
Web site: http://www.cancer.org

*National Cancer Institute (NCI).*    The National Cancer Institute (NCI) sponsors the Cancer Information Service (CIS), created to provide information and education about cancer and its treatments. CIS operates a toll-free telephone hotline in English and Spanish that offers excellent information in clear and easy to understand language on recent medical findings on cancer prevention and treatments, including some carefully prepared discussions of complementary and alternative approaches. The CIS can also refer you to local cancer programs and support services.

Address: Cancer Information Service
Building 31, Room 10A16
9000 Rockville Pike
Bethesda, MD 20892
Phone: 1-800-4-CANCER (1-800-422-6237)
Fax: 301-231-6941
Web site: http://www.nci.nih.gov/

The National Cancer Institute also sponsors Cancer Centers across the country. Hospitals and medical care complexes designated as Cancer Centers were selected based on their scientific eminence and their research approach. These hospitals receive grants from the NCI to further research efforts and offer clinical care. There are many excellent hospitals throughout the country, but if you are seeking treatment and one of these centers is an option, you may want to contact them. If you are not interested in receiving treatment, these Cancer Centers may still be helpful because they should be able to refer you to other cancer-related local resources. To find out the Cancer Center nearest to you or for further assistance in researching NCI's Cancer Centers, contact the NCI's Cancer Center Branch.

>Address:    Cancer Centers Branch
>            Office of the Deputy Director for Extramural Science
>            Executive Plaza North, Room 502, MSC 7383
>            6130 Executive Blvd.
>            Bethesda, MD 20892–7383
>            (for Express mail use Rockville, MD 20852)
>Phone:      301-496-8531
>Fax:        301-402-0181
>Web site:   http://www.nci.nih.gov/cancercenters

The *PDQ* (Physician Data Query) database is an additional NCI resource. It serves as a directory of

- Physicians who spend the majority of their time treating cancer patients (24,000 listings)
- Health care organizations that have organized programs of cancer care (2,500 listings)
- Mammography screening facilities (9,500 listings)

The PDQ is now including valuable information on some complementary and alternative therapies.

The PDQ database can be accessed in the following ways:

- CancerNet: PDQ information most likely to be sought by general public can be found at http://cancernet.nci.nih.gov
- Cancer Information Service: 1-800-4-CANCER, TTY 1-800-332-8615 (as listed above).
- PDQ Search Service: Free service that provides customized PDQ searches for health professionals who call 1-800-345-3300, fax 1-800-380-1575, or send an e-mail to pdqsearch@icicc.nci.nih.gov
- NCI's Information Associates Program (IAP): Full PDQ Internet access for IAP members who call 1-800-624-7890, fax 301-496-7600, or send an e-mail to iap@icicc.nci.nih.gov

- CancerFax: Free service for fax users can be accessed by
  1. Dialing 301-402-5874 on the handset of the Fax machine
  2. Requesting a contents list
  3. Entering a code number from the list that corresponds to the desired information
  4. Following the voice prompts to receive a faxed image of the information
- National Library of Medicine's (NLM) On-Line Access to scientific publications:

  *U.S.A.*

  MEDLARS, Medical Literature Analysis and Retrieval System, is available through medical or hospital libraries that have access to this system (maintained by the National Library of Medicine's computer network), An access code may be requested by contacting the MEDLARS Service Desk at 1-800-638-8480. There is a prorated charge of $18 an hour, with the typical search lasting only a few minutes.

  *Europe*

  Health care professionals in Europe can access the NLM On-Line through the European Organization for Research and Treatment of Cancer (EORTC).

  *Latin America and the Caribbean*

  NLM On-Line can be accessed through the academic network BITNET.

  - CD-ROM: Discs are sent out monthly on an annual subscription basis from commercial database distributors. Information on distributors can be obtained through Cancer Fax or the CancerNet Mail Service.
  - Publications: Free publications on specific issues can be downloaded from CancerNet or requested from CIS (see contact information above). For a list of publications, write to the NCI's Office of Cancer Communications, 31 Center Dr., MSC 2580, Bethesda, MD 20892-2580.

***National Coalition for Cancer Survivorship.*** The National Coalition for Cancer Survivorship is a patient-led organization that serves as an advocacy and resource group for people with cancer. It offers educational programs, support services, publications, and leadership in public policy issues that affect patients, such as health insurance and employment rights.

| | |
|---|---|
| Address: | 1010 Wayne Ave. |
| | Suite 505 |
| | Silver Springs, MD 20910-5600 |
| Phone: | 1-888-YES-NCCS (888-937-6227) |
| | or 301-650-8868 |
| Fax: | 301-565-9670 |
| E-mail: | info@cansearch.org |
| Web site: | http://www.cansearch.org |

## Integrative Medicine Resources

### CanHelp

- Personalized research and treatment information with interpretation of data for patient/client and for attending physician
- References and reports appropriate to patient/client's condition from CanHelp's files
- Synopsis of conversations concerning patient/client among CanHelp's medical advisor network

The founder and director, Patrick McGrady, does exhaustive research into both traditional and alternative/complementary medical options for the client's particular cancer situation. He then writes up his findings in an easy-to-understand format for non–medical professionals. Mr. McGrady also refers clients to practitioners with medical degrees and guides them away from treatments he feels are ineffective.

A full report is delivered to the client within one week of receipt of medical reports. The cost is $400 for U.S. clients, $250 for in-person consultation.

| | |
|---|---|
| Address: | 3111 Paradise Bay Rd. |
| | Port Ludlow, WA 98365-9771 |
| Phone: | 360-437-2291 |
| Fax: | 360-437-2272 |

### Patient-Directed Consultations

- Medical advice
- Information on treatment options (traditional and alternative)
- Physician-to-physician communication and advocacy on behalf of the patient/client

Dr. Renneker is a board-certified, university-affiliated family physician with training in most fields of medicine, including integrative (combining traditional/conservative treatment with alternative/complementary approaches). He works from within the medical establishment as a client advocate, doing "the work that the physicians would have liked to have done."

Dr. Renneker's advocacy and help in researching treatment options would be especially valuable for cases in which a diagnosis has not been reached, for rare illnesses, and for complicated medical situations.

Initial consultation by phone for 60 minutes is $250. Additional fees are based on a sliding scale from a minimum of $50 an hour to $300 an hour.

|  |  |
|---|---|
| Address: | Mark Renneker, M.D. |
|  | 4637 Ulloa St. |
|  | San Francisco, CA 94116 |
| Phone: | 415-681-5357 |
| Fax: | 415-681-9734 |
| E-mail: | renneker@well.com |

**The Moss Reports.** The Moss Reports service educates patients about the most promising alternative cancer treatments for their conditions. It is directed by Ralph W. Moss., Ph.D. A one-time fee of $297 includes an approximately 200-page report (which arrives in 2 to 3 days) and ongoing free updates. The report includes

- Specific and detailed recommendations about the best alternative cancer treatments for a specific diagnosis.
- Information about cutting-edge conventional treatment.

- Contact information for doctors, including those in one's region, whom Dr. Moss considers most expert in their fields.
- An international list of open-minded oncologists and expert alternative practitioners.

| | |
|---|---|
| **Address:** | **144 St. John's Place** |
| | **Brooklyn, NY 11217** |
| Phone: | 718-636-4433 |
| Fax: | 718-636-0186 |
| E-mail: | inquiries@cancerdecisions.com |
| Web site: | http://www.cancerdecisions.com |

## National Center for Complementary and Alternative Medicine

- Packet of information about current alternative cancer treatment studies
- Research funding for alternative medicine studies
- *Alternative Medicine: Expanding Medical Horizons* (428-page compendium of current alternative and complementary treatments)

The NCCAM functions as a clearinghouse and funding source for alternative medicine issues. Patients are encouraged to use NCCAM information if they are interested in presenting their oncologist with information about alternative and complementary approaches.

The packet of information is free. *Alternative Medicine* is free for medical and health professionals and $25 for others.

| | |
|---|---|
| Address: | P.O. Box 8218 |
| | Silver Spring, MD 20907 |
| Phone: | 888-644-6226 |
| Fax: | 301-495-4957 |
| Web site: | http://altmed.od.nih.gov |

## How to Find a Support Group

As previously discussed, we strongly recommend becoming involved in a support group. Many communities now have support groups. There are several approaches we recommend you take to find one in your area:

- Check your local newspaper. Newspapers are an excellent resource for finding out what is going on in your community—including support groups!
- Ask your physician if he or she is aware of any in the area. If the doctor is unable to help you, ask him or her to recommend someone for you to speak with who is familiar with these resources.
- Ask at your hospital or call other local hospitals. Many hospitals now have social services departments that either offer or can refer you to support groups and services in your area.
- Contact local churches, synagogues, or other religious centers. A growing number of churches and synagogues are offering support groups. Again, even if yours does not, they may be in touch with other places in the community that offer such services.
- Call your local branch of the American Cancer Society or a nearby Cancer Center sponsored by the National Cancer Institute. Not only do these organizations provide information, but they also can put you in contact with an excellent network of support groups and services in your area.
- Contact the American Self-Help Clearinghouse. This organization has a database that includes many support groups and state and regional self-help clearinghouses across the country. The American Self-Help Clearinghouse can refer you to groups it finds in its database and to a clearinghouse in your region. These state and regional clearinghouses have databases of local self-help groups and can direct you to groups in your community that address your needs. If the American Self-Help Clearinghouse can find no clearinghouse in your state, they will direct you to national cancer foundations that also refer to support groups. Additionally, the American Self-Help Clearinghouse provides information on virtually all the self-help groups in New Jersey, where they are housed. Their Web site is also an excellent resource.

|          |                          |
|----------|--------------------------|
| Address: | St. Clair's Health System |
|          | 25 Pocono Rd.            |
|          | Denville, NJ 07834       |
| Phone:   | 973-625-7101 or 973-625-9565 |
| Web site:| http://www.cmhc.com      |

The following organizations may also be helpful if you are seeking support groups or services:

*Cancer Care, Inc.*   Cancer Care, Inc. provides excellent services to cancer patients. Cancer Care runs a telephone hotline where oncology social workers offer counseling, educational materials, referrals to services in your community, and assistance in understanding medical information and issues. Cancer Care also sponsors support groups and educational programs; they have made great efforts to provide help to people who cannot attend these events in person by using teleconferencing to provide these educational programs and form telephone support groups. Cancer Care also has some excellent publications that you can order, free, including *A Helping Hand*, an outstanding resource guide that lists national and regional support, information, care, and advocacy organizations for cancer patients and their families.

|          |                          |
|----------|--------------------------|
| Address: | 1180 Avenue of the Americas |
|          | New York, NY 10036–3692  |
| Phone:   | 1-800-813-HOPE (1-800-813-4673) or |
|          | 212-719-0293             |
| E-mail:  | info@cancercare.org      |
| Web site:| http://www.cancercare.org |

*Cancer Hope Network.*   The Cancer Hope Network provides one-on-one support by matching people newly diagnosed with cancer with a trained volunteer cancer survivor. The Cancer Hope Network tries to connect you with a volunteer who may have had a similar experience, either by surviving the same type of cancer or undergoing similar treatment.

| | |
|---|---|
| **Address:** | **2 North Rd., Suite A** |
| | Chester, NJ 07930–2308 |
| Phone: | 1-877-HOPENET (1-877-467-3638) or |
| | 908-879-4039 |
| Fax: | 908-879-6518 |
| E-mail: | info@cancerhopenetwork.org |
| Web site: | http://www.cancerhopenetwork.org |

*Center for Attitudinal Healing.*    The Center for Attitudinal Healing is a safe place for individuals to reexamine their lives and overcome the fear, conflict, and separation that accompany personal crisis, whether that crisis is the result of illness, social conditions, or psychological trauma. The center has many years' experience working with children with life-threatening illnesses, including cancer. Programs based on the same philosophy and approach are available at other locations in the United States and abroad.

| | |
|---|---|
| Address: | 33 Buchanan Dr. |
| | Sausalito, CA 94965 |
| Phone: | 415-331-6161 |
| Fax: | 415-331-4545 |
| Web site: | http://www.healingcenter.org |

*Gilda's Club.*    A growing association of support centers in the United States named after the late comedian Gilda Radner, who died of ovarian cancer in 1989. The centers, or "Clubhouses," provide places where people with cancer and their families and friends join with others to build social and emotional support as a supplement to medical care. Free of charge and nonprofit, Gilda's Club offers support and networking groups, lectures, workshops, and social events in a nonresidential, homelike setting.

| | |
|---|---|
| **Address:** | **195 West Houston St.** |
| | New York, NY 10014 |
| Phone: | 212-647-9700 |
| Fax: | 212-647-1151 |
| Web site: | www.gildasclub.org |

*The Wellness Community.*    The Wellness Community is a national organization with centers across the county that provides free psychological and emotional support for cancer patients and their families. The Wellness Community network is based on the philosophy that the participation of cancer patients with their medical team is integral to the emotional well-being of the patient. At each of their locations the Wellness Community offers support groups for patients and their families, educational workshops and seminars on topics such as stress and pain management, yoga, *tai chi*, relaxation, and nutrition (led by experts in these fields), and social events. Contact their national office for more information or to find the Wellness Community nearest to you.

Address:　　35 East 7th St., Suite 412
　　　　　　　Cincinnati, OH 45202
Phone:　　　1-888-793-WELL (888-793-9355) or
　　　　　　　513-421-7111
Fax:　　　　513-421-7119
E-mail:　　　wellnessnational@fuse.net
Web site:　　http://www.wellnesscolumbus.org

*Organizations for Specific Cancers.* The following organizations focus on a particular type/types of cancer and either have branches across the country that offer support groups or can refer you to support groups in your area. These organizations can also be helpful by providing information on specific types of cancer. Please note that this list represents just a small sample of some of the better known organizations that provide support groups. There are many organizations that address other types of cancer and additional organizations that work with some of the most common cancers. Contact national organizations such as the ACS or CancerCare if you would like more information on support groups and services that will meet your particular needs.

Alliance for Lung Cancer Advocacy,
Support & Education (ALCASE)
Address:　　1601 Lincoln Ave.
　　　　　　　Vancouver, WA 98660
Phone:　　　1-800-298-2436 or 360-696-2436
E-mail:　　　info@alcase.org
Web site:　　http://www.teleport.com/~alcase

### American Brain Tumor Association (ABTA)

Address:    2720 River Rd., Suite 146
            Des Plaines, IL 60018
Phone:      1-800-886-2282 or 847-827-9910
E-mail:     abta@aol.com
Web site:   http://www.abta.org

### American Foundation for Urologic Disease (AFUD)

Address:    300 West Pratt St., Suite 401
            Baltimore, MD 21201
Phone:      1-800-828-7866 or 410-727-2908
E-mail:     admin@afud.org
Web site:   http://www.afud.org

### Candlelighters Childhood Cancer Foundation (CCCF)

Address:    7910 Woodmont Ave., Suite 460
            Bethesda, MD 20814-3015
Phone:      1-800-366-2223 or 301-657-8401
E-mail:     info@candlelighters.org
Web site:   http://www.candlelighters.org

### Encore Plus (breast and cervical cancer)

Address:    YWCA of the USA
            Office of the Women's Health Initiative
            624 Ninth St., NW
            Third Floor
            Washington, DC 20001
Phone:      1-800-95E-PLUS (1-800-953-7587) or
            202-628-3636
Fax:        202-783-7123
E-mail:     mcandreia@ywca.org
Web site:   http://www.ymcaencore.org

### International Myeloma Foundation (IMF)

Address:    2129 Stanley Hills Dr.
            Los Angeles, CA 90046
Phone:      1-800-452-CURE (1-800-452-2873) or
            213-656-1182
E-mail:     theimf@aol.com
Web site:   http://www.myeloma.org

### Leukemia Society of America (LSA)

Address:    600 Third Ave.
            New York, NY 10016

Phone:       1-800-955-4LSA (1-800-955-4572) or
             212-573-8484
E-mail:      infocenter@leukemia.org
Web site:    http://www.leukemia.org

**National Alliance of Breast Cancer Organizations (NABCO)**
Address:     9 East 37th St.
             10th Floor
             New York, NY 10016
Phone:       212-719-0154
E-mail:      nabcoinfo@aol.com
Web site:    http://www.nabco.org

**National Brain Tumor Foundation (NBTF)**
Address:     785 Market St., Suite 1600
             San Francisco, CA 94103
Phone:       1-800-934-CURE (1-800-934-2873) or
             415-284-0208
E-mail:      nbtf@braintumor.org
Web site:    http://www.braintumor.org

**National Lymphedema Network (NLN)**
Address:     2211 Post St., Suite 404
             San Francisco, CA 94115-3427
Phone:       1-800-541-3259 or 415-921-1306
E-mail:      nln@lymphnet.org
Web site:    http://www.lymphnet.org

**Post-Treatment Resource Program**
Address:     215 East 68th St., Ground Floor
             New York, NY 10021
Phone:       212-717-3527
E-mail:      zampinik@mskcc.org

**Support for People with Oral and
Head and Neck Cancer, Inc. (SPOHNC)**
Address:     P.O. Box 53
             Locust Valley, NY 11560-0053
Phone:       516-759-5333
E-mail:      info@spohnc.org
Web site:    http://www.spohnc.org

**US TOO International, Inc.** (Prostate Cancer)
Address:       930 North York Rd., Suite 50
               Hinsdale, IL 60521–2993
Phone:         1-800-808-7866 or 630-323-1002
E-mail:        uoa@deltanet.com
Web site:      http://www.ustoo.com

**Y-ME National Breast Cancer Organization**
Address:       212 West Van Buren St., 5th Floor
               Chicago, IL 60607-3908
Phone:         1-800-221-2141 (24-hour hotline) or
               312-986-8338 or 312-986-9505 (in Spanish)
E-mail:        info@yme.org
Web site:      http://www.y-me.org

## Other Support Services

*American Pain Society.*    The American Pain Society is a multidisciplinary educational and scientific organization working to serve people in pain. APS has a database of pain treatment centers and its members are associated with and can refer people to local centers.

Address:       4700 West Lake Ave.
               Glenview, IL 60025
Phone:         847-375-4715
Fax:           847-375-4777
E-mail:        info@ampainsoc.org
Web site:      http://www.ampainsoc.org

*Corporate Angel Network.*    The Corporate Angel Network provides air transportation to cancer patients and their families to and from cancer treatments free of charge. Transportation from the airport to the hospital and hotel accommodations can also sometimes be arranged. Participants must be able to walk unassisted and need no other special services. Flights are not always available, so alternate transportation plans must also be made.

Address:       Westchester County Airport
               Building One
               White Plains, NY 10604
Phone:         914-328-1313

Fax:          800-328-4226
E-mail:       info@corpangelnetwork.org
Web site:     http://www.corpangelnetwork.org

*National Patient Air Transport Hotline (NPATH).*  NPATH provides referrals for air travel services for patients who cannot afford transportation to attain necessary medical care.

Address:    P.O. Box 1940
            Manasses, VA 20108-0804
Phone:      800-296-1217 or 703-361-1191

*Women's Health Care Educational Network.*  The Women's Health Care Educational Network is a nonprofit organization made up of independent businesses that specialize in serving women who have had breast surgery. Information and referral services are provided for those seeking specialty items, such as wigs, maternity and nursing products, and compression products for lymphedoma.

Address:    Box 5061
            Tiffin, OH 44883
Phone:      800-991-8877
Fax:        419-448-5312

## RETREATS AND WELLNESS PROGRAMS
## FOR PEOPLE WITH CANCER

There are several residential wellness retreats throughout the country that specifically address the needs of cancer patients. Some of these are described below, followed by a list of other residential facilities that are designed to promote healthy living as well as provide a respite from daily stress.

*Commonweal Cancer Help Program (CCHP).*  The Commonweal Cancer Help Program was founded in 1985 by Michael Lerner, author of *Choices in Healing*, and has become a model for educational healing retreats for cancer patients. Commonweal is not a medical treatment program. Instead, Commonweal's week-long retreats aim to help cancer patients develop self-healing skills, offer information, and provide a nurturing environment for cancer patients seeking emotional and spiritual support. During Commonweal's retreats, participants learn techniques such as yoga, progressive relaxation, meditation, massage, and imagery to promote healing and stress reduction. The retreats include group therapy sessions; individual counseling; discussions on ways to integrate the arts into one's healing process; and guidance in making choices among mainstream, alternative, and complementary medicine. Meals are vegetarian. Retreats are limited to 8 people, and spouses and companions are invited to also attend at full fee. All participants must be under the care of an oncologist or other physician. Some scholarships are available. Commonweal also offers professional training programs to encourage other people to develop similar centers and can offer recommendations to people discouraged by Commonweal's substantial waiting list. Commonweal has worked directly with the Smith Farm Center for the Healing Arts' Cancer Help Program in Washington, D.C., and the Ting-Sha Institute in Point Reyes, California.

| | |
|---|---|
| Address: | P.O. Box 316 |
| | Bolinas, CA 94924 |
| Phone: | 415-868-0970 |
| Web site: | http://www.commonweal.org |

***Smith Farm Center for the Healing Arts.***   The Smith Farm Center for the Healing Arts was cofounded by Commonweal's president and founder Michael Lerner, and is designed to replicate this successful program. Smith Farm provides retreats on the East Coast that offer a similar structure and content to the retreats at Commonweal. Smith Farm also offers weekend workshops for physicians and other professionals on integrative approaches to healing, including programs for people interested in healing and the arts.

| | |
|---|---|
| Address: | Cancer Help Program |
| | 1229 15th St. NW |
| | Washington, DC 20005 |
| Phone: | 202-483-8600 |
| E-mail: | SmithFarm1@aol.com |
| Web site: | http://www.smithfarm.com |

*Ting-Sha Institute.*    The Ting-Sha Institute's proximity to Common-weal allows staff from Commonweal to also work at Ting-Sha's Cancer Help Programs. Ting-Sha offers week-long retreats for cancer patients that are similar to Commonweal's and also emphasize art, sensory awareness and movement (instead of yoga), and awakening to the present moment.

| | |
|---|---|
| Address: | **Cancer Help Retreats** |
| | **Box 226** |
| | **Port Reyes, CA 94956** |
| Phone: | 415-663-1190 |
| E-mail: | vv77@aol.com |
| Web site: | http://www.amacora.com/tingsha/ |
| | institutedescription.html |

The following three programs—Callanish Healing Retreats Society, Harmony Hill Cancer Retreats, and Hawaii Cancer Help Retreats—are among those listed on Commonweal's Web page as independent organizations that have received some degree of training or consultation from Commonweal staff.

### Callanish Healing Retreats Society

| | |
|---|---|
| Address: | #314–2902 West Broadway Ave. |
| | Vancouver, BC Canada |
| Phone: | 604-732-1012 |
| Fax: | 604-739-1800 |
| E-mail: | info@callanish.org |
| Web site: | http:// www.callanish.org |

Callanish retreats are open to people who have received a diagnosis of cancer and, if desired, their primary support person. Callanish was inspired by Commonweal and offers similar programming, including yoga, meditation, group counseling, massage, therapeutic touch, and creative exercises in art and music.

*Harmony Hill Cancer Retreats.*    Harmony Hill Cancer Retreats aim to create a place where people with cancer can examine and engage more deeply in their quest for meaning and the experience of living. Harmony Hill offers guests relaxation and meditation techniques, yoga, individual and group counseling, assistance in developing a plan for well-being, massage, and time to explore their creativity.

| | |
|---|---|
| **Address:** | **East 7362, Highway 106** |
| | Union, WA 98592 |
| Phone: | 360-898-2363 |
| E-mail: | harmonyh@halcyon.com |
| Web site: | http://www.harmonyhill.org |

*Hawaii Cancer Help Retreats.*   Hawaii Cancer Help Retreats are modeled after Commonweal's. They offer week-long retreats, with group and individual counseling and sessions in yoga, meditation, creativity, and alternative and complementary treatment options.

| | |
|---|---|
| **Address:** | **O Ka Mana Ka Ho'ola** |
| | P.O. Box 1236 |
| | Kamuela, HI 96743 |
| Phone: | 808-885-0995 or 808-885-7547 |

*Inner Mountain Wilderness Education Center.*   Alaska's powerful wilderness provides the Inner Mountain Wilderness Education Center with an amazing environment for its outdoor education programs for adult cancer survivors. These programs are intended to help cancer survivors to rebuild trust and confidence in their bodies by learning and engaging in outdoor activities such as rafting, sea-kayaking, backcountry hiking and camping, glacier travel, climbing, whale watching, bear spotting, and salmon fishing. They offer 5–10 day programs for groups of 8–12 participants. Their programs are not intended for people still undergoing treatment for cancer but rather for those in the later stages of recovery.

| | |
|---|---|
| **Address:** | **P.O. Box 123** |
| | Haines, AK 99827 |
| Phone/Fax: | 907-766-2074 |
| E-mail: | innermtn@kcd.com |
| Web site: | http://caseyd.meer.net/inner_mountain/ index2.htm |

*Other Spas and Wellness Programs.*   In addition to organizations that are designed for cancer patients and survivors, there are retreat centers and spas throughout the country that focus on holistic healing. Each has its own specialty and focus, so it is important to find one that matches your needs. When contacting the following organizations it is worth inquiring whether they have any retreats to specifically address the needs of people with cancer. Ask for reviews of their services from magazines and newspapers and feel comfortable asking to speak with former visitors. Before engaging in massage or any nutritional therapies these organizations may offer, it is important to check with your physician/healing practitioner to make sure the activities will not interfere with your current treatments.

One good way to find a spa or retreat appropriate for you is to contact Spa Finder, a free reservation service that creates and books spa vacation packages after helping you choose a spa that is right for you. The Web site has descriptions of many different retreats. Spa Finder also publishes a magazine that describes spas across the country (the cost of the magazine is redeemable when you book a spa through them).

> **Phone:** 1-800-ALL-SPAS (1-800-255-7727) toll-free
> or in New York City, 212-924-6800
> Web site: http://www.spafinders.com/

More generally, the Web can be a valuable resource in your search for a retreat. One site we recommend that has extensive listings (not specifically for people with cancer) is

> **The Consciousness Directory**
> Web site: http://www.thecd.com/retreats/

The following specific wellness retreats and spas have fine reputations. Some are more costly than others and each has its own particular focus, so call for a brochure or browse their Web pages to decide whether any of these places meets your needs.

> **The Chopra Center for Well Being**
> Located in: La Jolla, CA
> Phone: 1-888-424.6772 or 619-551-7788
> Fax: 619-551-7811
> E-mail: info@chopra.com
> Web site: http://www.chopra.com/ccwbwelcome.htm

### The Esalen Institute
Located in:    Big Sur, CA
Phone:         408-667-3000
Web site:      http://www.esaleninstitute.com

### Green Gulch Farm Zen Center
Located in:    Sausalito, CA
Phone:         415-383-3134
Web site:      http://www.sfzc.com

### Insight Meditation Society
Located in:    Barre, MA
Phone:         978-355-4378
Web site:      http://www.dharma.org

### Kripalu Center for Yoga and Health
Located in:    Lenox, MA
Phone:         1-800-741-7353 or 413-637-3280
Web site:      http://www.vgernet.net/kali/entrance.html

### Omega Institute of Holistic Studies
Located in:    Rhineback, NY
Phone:         1-800-944-1001
Web site:      http://www.omega-inst.org

### The Raj
Located in:    Fairfield, IA
Phone:         1-800-248-9050
Web site:      http://www.theraj.com

### Tassajara Zen Mountain Monastery
Located in:    San Francisco, CA
Phone:         415-431-3771
Web site:      http://www.zendo.com/~sfzc

There are also nonresidential programs designed to teach mind-body skills to cancer patients. The headquarters of the following two programs are both in Massachusetts, but each has program affiliates and can offer referrals in other parts of the country.

### Beth Israel Deaconess Medical Center

| | |
|---|---|
| Address: | Division of Behavioral Medicine and the Mind-Body Medical Institute |
| | 110 Francis St., Suite 1A |
| | Boston, MA 02215 |
| Phone: | 617-632-9530 |
| Fax: | 617-632-7383 |

The Beth Israel Deaconess Medical Center offers 9-week outpatient groups for people with cancer, teaching mind-body techniques based on Dr. Herbert Benson's work with the "relaxation response." The practices taught are intended to help patients cope with the stress and pain of illness as well as to enhance their capacity for self-healing.

### University of Massachusetts Memorial Health Center

| | |
|---|---|
| Address: | Stress Reduction Clinic/ Center for Mindfulness |
| | Shaw Building |
| | 55 Lake Ave., North |
| | Worcester, MA 01655 |
| Phone: | 508-856-2656 |
| Fax: | 508-856-1977 |

The 8-week courses offered at the Stress Reduction Clinic teach people with chronic illness mindfulness meditation and yoga and help participants deal with pain, stress, and the challenge of taking care of oneself. These courses are based on the work of its director, Jon Kabat-Zinn. Participants need a physician's referral to join the course.

## FINDING AN ALTERNATIVE HEALTH PRACTITIONER

There are several ways to find alternative or complementary practitioners or classes. We suggest the following methods to find one in your community:

- Begin by asking your physician for referrals. Increasingly, responsible physicians are developing firsthand knowledge of local practitioners and are making referrals just as they would to other medical specialists.
- Ask those you trust—family and friends—for recommendations. Word of mouth remains one of the best sources of information.
- Look in your local yellow pages or the yellow pages for the nearest major city. Most yellow pages now include listings for alternative and complementary health practitioners such as acupuncturists, chiropractors, massage therapists, meditation instructors, and yoga teachers.
- Find out if your community has an alternative health or new age directory or journal. Alternative and complementary health practitioners often are listed or are advertised in these sources.
- Check adult education classes near you. Complementary approaches such as yoga, meditation, and nutrition are being offered in increasing numbers through classes in many communities.
- Call your local gym or health club. Some now offer classes in areas such as nutrition and yoga, and even if they do not, they may be able to direct you to organizations that do or may be familiar with health practitioners in the area.
- Find directories on the Web. Several of the alternative health sites described in Appendix B have directories of alternative health practitioners online.
- Contact a national umbrella organization. The following organizations have directories of alternative and complementary health practitioners.

### Biofeedback

**Biofeedback Certification Institute of America**
Address:    10200 West 44th Ave., Suite 304
            Wheatridge, CO 80033
Phone:      303-420-2902

## Herbal Medicine

**America Herbalists Guild**
Address:     P.O. Box 70
             Roosevelt, UT 84066
Phone:       435-722-8434
Web site:    http://www.healthy.net/herbalists

**American Botanical Council**
Address:     P.O. Box 201660
             Austin, TX 78720
Phone:       512-331-8868

## Holistic Medicine

**American Holistic Medical Association**
Address:     6728 Old McLean Village Dr.
             McLean, VA 22101-3906
Phone:       703-556-9728
Web site:    http://www.holisticmedicine.org

**American Holistic Nurses' Association**
Address:     4101 Lake Boone Trail, Suite 201
             Raleigh, NC 27607
Phone:       800-278-AHNA
Fax:         919-787-4916

## Homeopathy

**National Center for Homeopathy**
Address:     801 North Fairfax St., Suite 306
             Alexandria, VA 22134
Phone:       703-548-7790
Web site:    http://homeopathic.org

## Hypnosis

**American Society of Clinical Hypnosis**
Address:     2200 East Devon Ave., Suite 291
             Des Plaines, IL 60018
Phone:       708-297-3317

**Milton Erickson Foundation**

Address:    3606 North 24th St.
Phoenix, AZ 85016

Phone:    602-956-6196

## Imagery

**Academy for Guided Imagery**

Address:    P.O. Box 2070
Mill Valley, CA 94942

Phone:    800-726-2070

## Meditation

**Insight Meditation Society and the
Barre Center for Buddhist Studies**

Address:    149 Lockwood Rd.
Barre, MA 01005

Phone:    978-355-2347

Fax:    978-355-2798

Web site:    http://www.dharma.org

## Massage and Bodywork

**American Massage Therapy Association**

Address:    820 Davis St., Suite 100
Evanston, IL 60201-4444

Phone:    708-864-0123

## Nutrition

**American Dietetic Association**

Address:    216 West Jackson, Suite 800
Chicago, IL 60606

Phone:    312-899-0040

Web site:    http://www.eatright.org/

## Therapeutic Touch

**Nurse Healers Professional Associates, Inc.**

Address:    175 Fifth Ave.
New York, NY 10010

Phone:    212-886-3776

## *Traditional Chinese Medicine*

### American Academy of Medical Acupuncture
Address:    5820 Wilshire Blvd., Suite 500
Los Angeles, CA 90036
Phone:    213-937-5514
Web site:    http://www.medicalacupuncture.org

### American Association of Oriental Medicine
Address:    433 Front St.
Catasauqua, PA 18032
Phone:    610-266-1433
Web site:    http://www.aaom.org

### Institute for Traditional Medicine
Address:    2017 S.E. Hawthorne
Portland, OR 97214
Phone:    503-233-4907
Web site:    http://www.itmonline.org

# Appendix B
# Guide to
# Internet Resources

## Introduction

The Internet is an important resource, providing an astounding quantity and diversity of information at great speed and with relative ease. It is an extremely useful tool to gather information and to connect, literally around the world, with a support network.

The Internet is an excellent place to learn more about one's diagnosis and treatment options. Many well-known organizations aiming to help cancer patients, such as the National Cancer Institute, have sites on the World Wide Web (WWW) that offer information about specific illnesses. There are also Web sites developed by individuals that provide extensive information about cancer and its treatments. In addition to presenting information, these sites often have excellent suggestions for finding further sources of information and support. As anyone who has ever undertaken a research project knows, one of the hardest steps to getting the information you need is knowing where to look. The creators of these sites have already done this groundwork, simplifying and expediting one's search.

A few cautionary notes as you begin to research: As the best sites comment, information attained over the Internet should not replace seeing a physician or healer. While the knowledge one can gain through research on the Internet can be a great asset to effective communication between patient and doctor, it is not meant to displace this important partnership. Second, the Internet offers anonymity that allows anyone to create a Web site or pose as a healer or physician. As always, use your best judgment in evaluating the information people offer, keeping in mind that you do not know who these people are. Be particularly mindful of anyone who's trying to sell you something, is extremely aggressive in promoting an approach—especially to the exclusion of other treatments—or whose claims are not backed by scientific evidence. While these caveats should not dissuade you from freely exploring sites, it is important to stay alert as you navigate. Finally, share the information with someone—ideally an open-minded physician—who can help you critique and evaluate what you have found out.

Not everyone wants to do research on the Internet, and it is important to remember that one can still research effectively without using this tool. However, if you want to do research on the Internet but do not own a computer or feel uncomfortable navigating the Web, do not worry. You can still use the Internet for research; you just need to find out how.

## Access to Computers and the Internet

If you do not own a computer, you can probably find one available for public use. Your local library or any university library should have computers with access to the Internet. Even if they do not, they may be able to direct you to one. You may also want to contact your local hospital. Some have a patient advocate's office that should be able to help you in your search. Computer repair people and merchants are also often well informed as to local computer resources. Finally, it is likely you have a friend or an acquaintance who does have a computer. Start asking around and you might find someone who would be willing to let you use his or her computer for your research.

If you do not feel comfortable navigating the Internet, but have access to a computer, one of the best ways to begin your research is with the help of someone who is familiar with the Internet. Contacting any of the resources mentioned above is a good way to find someone to help you. For instance, by calling your local college or high school computer lab, you may be able to find a student who would volunteer or for a small fee show you the basics of Internet research or work with you to gather information. Community and religious organizations may also be aware of people in your neighborhood who would be happy to help. In many areas, adult education computer classes are available. You may want to contact the instructors of these courses to see if one of them would give you a lesson.

## Finding Information

To begin your search, it may be helpful to read over the following sites that offer guidance on how to utilize the Internet for cancer research.

> **CanSearch**
> http://www.cansearch.org

Designed by the National Coalition of Cancer Survivorship, CanSearch is a wonderful guide through cancer resources on the Internet. CanSearch takes you step-by-step through the online research process, helping you to navigate and connect to the vast number of cancer resources identified by the coalition.

> **Complementary and Alternative Medicine (CAM)**
> Resources for Cancer Research on the World Wide
> Web (WWW)
> http://cpmcnet.columbia.edu/dept/rosenthal/cam.html

This site presents an organized approach to beginning online research for CAM treatments for cancer on the Web. In addition to providing links to helpful resources, it offers advice on how to evaluate sites that claim to have treatment options.

### General Information

The Web sites below are ones that we have found to be particularly helpful in the initial steps of cancer research. Although this list is by no means exhaustive, these sites provide a good place from which to begin your search.

> **American Cancer Society**
> http://www.cancer.org

The American Cancer Society gives information on specific types of cancer, lists a variety of local resources for cancer patients and their families by state, and provides daily news updates on the latest developments in cancer research.

### CancerGuide
http://www.cancerguide.org

Steve Dunn, a former cancer patient, has created CancerGuide to assist other patients in their journey. At first glance, Dunn's site may appear less comprehensive than those produced by larger institutions, but there actually is a great deal of excellent information. Dunn's site emphasizes patient's stories and thoughtful articles; be sure to read Stephen Jay Gould's essay, "The Median Isn't the Message," when visiting this site. Dunn also provides top-notch sections on unconventional and alternative therapies—his advice on evaluating alternative therapies and his links to information on specific alternative treatments are particularly helpful.

### CancerNet
http://cancernet.nci.nih.gov/

The U.S. National Cancer Institute's (NCI) CancerNet is an excellent source of information. One of CancerNet's best features is the Physician's Data Query (PDQ), a database that contains peer-reviewed summaries on cancer screening, prevention, treatment, and care; timely and extensive information on clinical trials, some of which are still ongoing; and a directory of physicians, genetic counselors, and organizations that specialize in cancer care. CancerNet also features CancerLit, a bibliographic database of the National Library of Medicine, which offers records and abstracts of many articles. Also extremely helpful is CancerNet's cancerTrials database, which offers in-depth information on the latest clinical trials.

### Guide to Internet Resources for Cancer
http://www.ncl.ac.uk/~nchwww/guides/clinks1.htm

The University of Newcastle and the North of England Children's Cancer Research Unit's (NECCRU) Guide to Internet Resources for

Cancer provides links to information on specific types of cancer; an important section on "Quality of Medical Information on the Internet"; international resources, and an extensive list of support groups, mailing lists, and chat rooms. This site's design is somewhat confusing; while it is good to start at the homepage (Web site address above), you can also go directly to the patient's public menu at http://www.ncl.ac.uk/~nchwww/guides/clinks6.htm#menu, which provides access to many of the features of this guide.

**OncoLink**
http://cancer.med.upenn.edu

OncoLink, from the University of Pennsylvania's Cancer Center, is a thorough and helpful site with information on a wide variety of topics, including psychosocial support, clinical trials, cancer prevention, causes and screening, medical supportive care, and financial issues.

**Yahoo!**
http://www.yahoo.com/Health/Diseases_and_
Conditions/cancer

Yahoo offers information on specific types of cancer, references to helpful institutes, journals, organizations, and an extensive listing of links to other cancer resources and support groups on the Web.

## Alternative and Complementary Medicine

As previously noted, many of the sites listed above have sections on complementary and alternative medicine (CAM). The following sites focus specifically on CAM and are well worth visiting when exploring these treatment options.

**Alternative Health News Online**
http://www.altmedicine.com/

Alternative Health News Online contains a great deal of helpful information, including timely news articles and health updates; a search engine for its own Web site and links to other search engines;

and extensive information on CAM treatments such as nutrition, mind-body methods, and traditional chinese medicine.

**The Alternative Medicine Homepage**
http://www.pitt.edu/~cbw/altm.html

The Alternative Medicine Homepage offers a general overview of alternative therapies, including links to alternative medicine databases, Web sites, government and practitioner directories, and on-line mailing lists.

**Ask NOAH (New York Online Access to Health)**
http://www.noah.cuny.edu/alternative/alternative.html

Ask NOAH's alternative health page is divided into three sections: comprehensive information on many alternative care modalities, resource directories, and disease and health concerns.

**Gerson Research Organization**
http://www.gerson-research.org

This Web site focuses on Dr. Max Gerson's diet-based cancer therapy. A profile of the Gerson therapy and related articles are accessible.

**HealthWorld Online**
http://www.healthy.net

This online health resource center offers information on a great deal of wellness topics, including nutrition, fitness, self-care, guided imagery, and alternative treatments. It also has a section on "diseases and conditions" that provides specific information about cancer prevention and treatment. If you visit this site, note that while some of the Web sites suggested are strictly informative, others are commercial.

**Kushi Institute: macrobioticsOnline**
http://www.macrobiotics.org

The Kushi Institute promotes health through the macrobiotic diet. Its Web page includes case histories, articles, recipes, and information on Kushi Institute programs. The site also hosts an online supplies catalog of organic whole-foods, cookware, and a large selection of books.

**Mining Co. Guide to Alternative Therapy**
http://altmedicine.miningco.com/

This guide to alternative medicine provides links to different CAM modalities and a few articles pertaining directly to cancer treatments. One of this site's best links is to http://www.bu.edu/CO-HIS/cancer/about/alttx/alttherp.htm, a site produced by Boston University Medical Center that contains comprehensive descriptions of many alternative treatments for cancer.

**National Institutes of Health: National Center for Complementary and Alternative Medicine**
http://altmed.od.nih.gov/nccam/

The National Center for Complimentary and Alternative Medicine (NCCAM) was created to research and distribute information on complementary and alternative medicine. Research grants have allowed further exploration of these therapies, including work on cancer treatments at the University of Texas (see below). The NCCAM Web site offers information on the center's projects and program areas. It also includes a listing of issues to consider before trying CAM, answers to frequently asked questions about CAM, an overview of different CAM practices, and a very helpful "Citation Index" comprising articles from the National Library of Medicine's Medline database.

**People Against Cancer**
http://www.dodgenet.com/nocancer

People Against Cancer is a nonprofit organization that distributes educational materials on alternative cancer therapies. Its Web page profiles the organization's services.

**University of Texas Center for Alternative Medicine Research in Cancer**
http://www.sph.uth.tmc.edu/utcam/

The University of Texas Center for Alternative Medicine Research, a research institute supported by the National Center for Complementary and Alternative Medicine and the National Cancer Institute, was established to evaluate CAM cancer treatments. Its Web site is excellent, describing research projects underway at the center and providing an extensive listing of additional CAM resources including books, periodicals, Web sites, and organizations.

## Medical Articles

The Internet is also an excellent way to find medical articles. There are databases designed to search medical journals on specific topics. It is important to remember that these medical articles are written for doctors and can be extremely difficult to understand. If you do find an article that seems relevant but are having a hard time deciphering the medical language, you can ask your doctor to look at it with you.

CancerNet, as previously described, is an excellent place to obtain abstracts of articles on cancer-related topics.

> **MedLine**
> http://www.nlm.nih.gov/

If you are looking for a wider range of medical topics, MedLine, another database of the National Library of Medicine, provides references to published articles in over 3,900 medical journals. The National Institutes of Health's National Center for Complementary and Alternative Medicine (NCCAM) recommends using MedLine to search for articles on complementary and alternative treatments (CAM). Go to http://altmed.od.nih.gov/nccam/resources/cam-ci/ for NCCAM's guide to using MedLine to search for information on CAM. You can find abstracts of these and other articles through either of two search engines, PubMed or Internet Grateful Med. Internet Grateful Med also has a feature that allows you to search for related articles for any abstract you have found.

Another way to find articles is by searching directly in a particular medical journal. The journals listed here are professional and well known. Several of these sources allow you to access only the abstracts of articles. However, should you want more information, you can usually order the full text for a fee.

**Alternative Therapies in Health and Medicine**
http://www.alternative-therapies.com

**British Medical Journal**
http://www.bmj.com

**The Journal of Chinese Medicine**
http://www.pavilion.co.uk/jcm/

**Journal of Clinical Oncology**
http://www.jco.org

**The Journal of the American Medical Association**
http://www.jama.com

**The Journal of Alternative and Complementary Medicine**
http://www.liebertpub.com

**M. D. Anderson Oncology**
http://www.mdacc.tmc.edu/~oncolog

**New England Journal of Medicine**
http://www.nejm.org/content/index.asp

**HealthNotes.com**
http://www.nprc.com

## Books

There are many informative books on cancer, including the ones we have listed in our bibliography. The Web can be utilized as a means to sort through and find the most relevant books for one's research. Companies like Amazon.com., which sell books online, have useful features such as summaries of books, reviews, and additional recommended titles on related topics, which can facilitate one's search for helpful literature.

**amazon.com**
http://www.amazon.com

## Mailing Lists and Chat Rooms

The Internet allows people from all over the world to connect online and utilize each other as sources of information and support. As discussed, we strongly recommend finding an in-person support group. Ideally, one could use online communication as an additional form of emotional support. However, for some people, because of obstacles such as their location, the Internet may be a primary means to communicate with other people who are surviving cancer. It also may be one of the only ways to find a group of people with one's specific type of cancer. For everyone, whatever other resources are available, the Internet offers a place where people can connect 24 hours a day, 7 days a week, from any location. Communicating with other patients can provide comfort as well as extensive information from others who are researching and learning about cancer and its treatments. There are several ways to find people online who want to communicate about cancer and its effects. The most common and useful are mailing lists and chat rooms.

### Mailing Lists

Perhaps the most helpful way to communicate with others on the Internet is through mailing lists. People subscribe to mailing lists to discuss a particular topic by using e-mail. All mail is sent to one address and is then automatically sent to all subscribers of the mailing list. Some of you may have heard the term "listserv"; this is another name for a mailing list and refers to the computer program that distributes mail and maintains a list of subscribers.

People who participate in cancer mailing lists exchange information with and provide support to one another. Although most mailing lists for cancer patients do not have active "moderators" who intervene in conversations, they all have "listowners" who supervise the mailing list. The listowners often establish rules of etiquette and appropriateness and make sure new members receive this information. They can watch out for subscribers sending unsuitable messages and eliminate someone from the list who is not abiding by proper codes of conduct. The listowner's role helps to minimize ad vertising and messages intended to be hostile. The format of a mailing list, in which each person receives all mail sent by other subscribers, seems more conducive to creating supportive relationships between members than other forms of Internet communication. Mailing lists are very popular, so expect your mail volume to increase significantly when subscribing to a list.

One of the easiest ways to find a mailing list to join is to go to visit the Web site of the Association of On-Line Cancer Resources (ACOR). This organization sponsors many mailing lists on cancer and also provides links to support groups, articles by cancer survivors, and access to CancerNet and medical abstracts.

> **Association of On-Line Cancer Resources**
> http://www.medinfo.org/listserv.html

Many Web sites on cancer also suggest appropriate mailing lists, so when visiting these sites, it is worth seeing if there are any recommendations. One of the best of these is OncoLink, which provides an "Automated E-mail List Subscriber Form" that allows you to directly subscribe to mailing lists (many of which are sponsored by ACOR) from the site.

> **OncoLink**
> http://www.oncolink.upenn.edu/forms/listserv.html

Another helpful site on which to find mailing lists is LISZT, an extensive database of mailing lists including, but not specific to, cancer-related lists.

> **LISZT**
> http://www.liszt.com

### Chat Rooms

Chat rooms are specific "places" designated on the Internet where people can correspond with each other in "real time." Messages appear on one's computer screen as they are typed, allowing people to have online conversations. While some people enjoy the immediacy and more direct communication chat rooms offer, they are also a less reliable form of correspondence than mailing lists or newsgroups because communication is limited to conversations with whoever happens to be visiting the chat room at the same time you are. Further, chat rooms are not monitored and can attract people trying to take advantage of others. Different Web servers have their own chat rooms. Many of these servers allow you to establish your own chat space on a particular topic. Depending on what kind of server you have, this process will be slightly different.

Another way to access chat rooms is through Internet Relay Chat (IRC), which allows people with different servers to converse by connecting through IRC's network. Conversations on IRC can be public or private. For more information on IRC, go to http://www.irchelp.org/. IRC is composed of many different "channels" on a variety of topics; the most popular for cancer patients is OncoChat. To access IRC's OncoChat, go to http://www.oncochat.org/index.html.

Despite the Internet's limitations and the cautiousness we recommend when exploring online communication, many people have received enormous support and extremely helpful information and guidance from the online relationships they have formed.

# Notes

## Introduction

p. xiii    **renegade cell:** Weinberg, R.A. 1998. *One Renegade Cell: How Cancer Begins.* New York: Basic Books.

## Chapter 1: In the Beginning. . .

p. 5    **Norman Cousins:** Cousins, Norman. 1979. *Anatomy of an Illness.* New York: W.W. Norton and Company.

p. 8    **Steven Greer, M.D.:** Greer, S., Morris, T., Pettingale, K. W. 1979. "Psychological Response to Breast Cancer: Effect on Outcome." *Lancet.* 2(8146):785–787.

Greer, S. 1989. "Can Psychological Therapy Improve the Quality of Life of Patients with Cancer?" *British Journal of Cancer.* 59(4):149–151.

Greer, S., et al. 1990. "Psychological Response to Breast Cancer and 15-year Outcome." *Lancet.* 335(8680):49–50.

Greer, S. 1991. "Psychological Response to Cancer and Survival." *Psychological Medicine.* 21:43–49.

Greer, S., et al. 1991. "Evaluation of Adjuvant Psychological Therapy for Clinically Referred Cancer Patients?" *British Journal of Cancer.* 63:257–260.

p. 10    **a study by Greer's collaborators:** Watson, M., et al. 1999. "Influence of Psychological Response on Survival in Breast Cancer: A Population-Based Cohort Study." *Lancet.* 354: 1331–1336.

Temoshok, L. 1987. "Personality, Coping Style, Emotion and Cancer: Towards an Integrative Model." *Cancer Surveys.* 6(3):545–567.

p. 13    **Psychologist James Pennebaker:** Pennebaker, J. W. 1993. "Putting Stress into Words: Health, Linguistic, and Therapeutic Implications." *Behavioral Research and Therapy.* 31(6):539–548.

Pennebaker, J. W., et al. 1990. "Accelerating the Coping Process." *Journal of Personality and Social Psychology.* 58(3): 528–537.

p. 16     **work of Suzanne Kobasa Ouellette:** Kobasa, S. C. 1982. "Commitment and Coping in Stress Resistance Among Lawyers." *Journal of Personality and Social Psychology.* 42(4):707–717.
Kobasa, S. C. 1979. "Stressful Life Events, Personality, and Health: An Inquiry into Hardiness." *Journal of Personality and Social Psychology.* 37:1–11.

p. 17     **study by Ellen Langer and Judith Rodin:** Langer, E. J., Rodin, J. 1976. "The Effects of Choice and Enhanced Personal Responsibility for the Aged: A Field Experiment in an Institutional Setting." *Journal of Personality and Social Psychology.* 34: 191–198.

## Chapter 2: Facts for Life

p. 21     **NCI statistics:** 1998 Factbook, Cancer Stattistics on the National Cancer Institute's Web site is www.nci.nih.gov.

p. 21     **ACS statistics:** 1998 Factbook and Figures: Selected Cancers, the American Cancer Society's Web site is www.cancer.org.

p. 25     **Dr. Robert Weinberg:** Weinberg, R. A. 1998. *One Renegade Cell: How Cancer Begins.* New York: Basic Books.

p. 29     **she was confused by what her doctors tried to tell her:** "Many Patients Said to Leave Their MD's Office Without Understanding What They've Been Told." *Oncology.* 9(11):1134.

p. 33     **struggle with technical information:** Brody, J. E. August 11, 1998. "A Study Guide to Scientific Studies." *New York Times.* C7.
Hibbard, J., et al. 1997. "Informing Consumer Decisions in Health Care: Implications from Decision-Making Research." *Milbank Quarterly.* 75(3):395–415.
Riegelman, R. K., Hirsch, R. P. 1996. *Studying a Study and Testing a Test,* 3rd ed. New York: Little, Brown and Company.

p. 34     **how probability applies:** Goodman, S. N. September 27, 1998. "The Capability of Probability." *Washington Post.* Outlook/C3.

p. 39     **Harvard paleontologist Stephen Jay Gould:** Gould, Stephen Jay. *Bully for Brontosaurus: Reflections in Natural History.* New York: W.W.Norton and Company, 1991.

p. 40     **resources on history of medicine:** Ackerknecht, E.A. *A Short History of Medicine,* (rev. ed.). Baltimore:Johns Hopkins Univ. Press, 1982.
Cassedy, J.H. *Medicine in America: A Short History.* Baltimore: Johns Hopkins Univ. Press, 1991.
Golub, E.S. *The Limits of Medicine: How Science Shapes Our Hope for the Cure.* New York: Times Books, 1994.

Sigerist, H.E. *A History of Medicine.* New York: Oxford Univ. Press, 1987; originally published in 1951.

p. 44    **"best case series":** Information on "The NCI Best Case Series Process" can be found on the Center for Mind-Body Medicine's web site, located at www.cmbm.org in the 1999 Comprehensive Cancer Care (CCC) transcripts.

p. 46    **use studies in different ways:** Payer, Lynn: *Medicine and Culture.* New York; Holt, 1988.

p. 48    **Marilyn Schlitz:** Braud, W., Schlitz, M. 1992. "Consciousness Interactions with Remote Biological Systems: Anomalous Intentionality Effects." *Subtle Energies.* 2(1):1–46.

Information presented by Dr. Schlitz can be found in the 1998 CCC transcripts titled "Remarkable Recovery" at www.cmbm.org.

## Chapter 3: Mind-Body Medicine

p. 55    **endocrine and immune systems:** Pert, C. and Harris Dienstfrey. 1988. "The Neuropeptide Network." *Annals of the New York Academy of Sciences.* Vol. 521.

Pert, Candace. *Molecules of Emotion.* New York: Scribner, 1997.

p. 55    **share a common chemical language:** Maier, S. F. & Watkins, L. R. 1998. "Cytokines for Psychologists: Implications of Bidirectional Immune-to-Brain Communication for Understanding Behavior, Mood and Cognition." *Psychological Review.* 105(1):83–107.

p. 55    **Walter Bradford Cannon :** Cannon, W.B. *The Wisdom of the Body.* New York: W.W. Norton, 1926.

p. 56    **Selye and "the general adaptation syndrome":** Selye, H. *The Stress of Life.* New York: McGraw-Hill, 1956.

p. 57    **Meyer Friedman and Ray Rosenman:** Freidman, M. & Rosenman, R.H. *Type A Behavior and Your Heart.* New York: Knopf, 1974.

p. 57    **repressed hostility is the primary culprit:** Williams, R. *The Trusting Heart.* New York: Times Books, 1989.

p. 58    **George Solomon at Stanford:** Solomon G.F. "Emotions Immunity and Disease," in L. Temoshok et al., eds., *Emotion in Health and Illness.* New York: Grune and Stratton, 1983.

p. 58    **Robert Ader and David Felten:** Ader, R., Felten, D.L. & Cohen, N. eds. *Psychoneuroimmunology,* second edition. San Diego: Academic Press, 1991.

p. 58    **Candace Pert and Solomon Snyder:** Pert, Candace. *Molecules of Emotion.* New York: Scribner, 1997.

p. 59    **Claus Bahnson reviewed the literature:** Bahnson, C.B. 1980. "Stress and Cancer: The State of the Art." *Psychosomatics.* 21(12):975.

p. 59    **Caroline Thomas' thirty-year study:** Thomas, C. B. & Duszynski, K. R. 1974. "Closeness to Parents and the Family Constellation in a Prospective Study of Five Disease States: Suicide, Mental Illness, Malignant Tumor, Hypertension, and Coronary Heart Disease." *Hopkins Med. J.* 134:251–70.

p. 59    **Schmale and Spence's observations:** Bahnson, C.B. 1980. "Stress and Cancer: The State of the Art." *Psychosomatics.* 21(12):975.

p. 59    **LeShan's and Worthington's findings:** LeShan, L. 1994. *Cancer as a Turning Point, Revised Edition.* New York: Penguin Group.
LeShan, L. 1991. "A New Question in Studying Psychosocial Interventions and Cancer." *Journal of Personality and Social Psychology.* 61:899–909.

p. 60    **stress of a variety of kinds can decrease immune functioning:** Jemmott, J. B., et al. 1983. "Academic Stress, Power Motivation, and Decrease in Secretion Rate of Salivary Secretory Immunoglobin A." *Lancet.* June 25:1,400–2.
Pike, J.L, et al. 1997. "Chronic Life Stress Alters Sympathetic , Neuroendocrine, and Immune Responsivity to an Acute Pschological Stressor in Humans." *Psychosom Med.* Jul-Aug; 59(4): 447–57.

p. 60    **impairing the effectiveness of DNA repair:** Kiecolt-Glaser J.K., et al. 1985. "Distress and DNA Repair in Human Lymphocytes." *Journal of Behavioral Medicine.* 89(4):311–320.

p. 60    **stress from which they have been unable to escape:** Laudenslager, Mark L. 1983. "Coping and Immunosuppression: Inescapable but Not Escapable Shock Suppresses Lymphocyte Proliferation." *Science.* 221: 568–570.

p. 60    **"repressive coping" style:** Greer, S., Watson, M. 1985. "Towards a Psychobiological Model of Cancer: Psychological Considerations." *Social Science and Medicine* 20(8):773–77.
Temoshek, L. 1987. "Personality, Coping Style, Emotion and Cancer: Towards an Integrative Model." *Cancer Surveys.* 6(3):545–566.

p. 60    **the association is at best a *weak* one:** McKenna, M. C., et al. 1999. "Psychosocial Factors and the Development of Breast Cancer: A Meta-Analysis." *Health Psychology.* 18(5):52–61.
Watson M., et al. 1999. "Influence of Psychological Response on Survival in Breast Cancer: A Population-Based Cohort Study." *Lancet.* 354: 1331–1336.

p. 60    **Bernard Fox:** Fox, B. H. 1995. "The Role of Psychological Factors in Cancer Incidence and Prognosis." *Oncology.* 9(3):245–253.

Fox, B. H. 1999. "Mind-Body Research in Psychooncology: Where do we go from here?" *Advances in Mind-Body Medicine* 15:264–266.

p. 62    **"quality of life" studies:** Buccheri, G. F., Ferrigno D., Tamburnini, M., Brunelli C. 1995. "The Patient's Perception of His Own Quality of Life Might Have an Adjunctive Prognostic Significance in Lung Cancer" *Lung Cancer.* 12(1–2):45–58.

Coates, A., Gebsk, V., Signorini, D., et al. 1992. "Prognostic Value of Quality of Life Scores During Chemotherapy for Advanced Breast Cancer." *Journal of Clinical Oncology.* 10(1):833–838.

Ganz, P. A., Kee, J. J., Diau, J. 1991. "Quality of Life Assessment: An Independent Prognostic Variable for Survival in Lung Cancer." *Cancer.* 67(3):131–135.

p. 62    **Greer and his colleagues' work on coping:** Greer, S., Morris, T., Pettingale, K. W. 1979. "Psychological Response to Breast Cancer: Effect on Outcome." *Lancet.* 2(8146):785–787.

Greer, S., et al. 1990. "Psychological Response to Breast Cancer and 15-year Outcome." *Lancet.* 335(8680):49–50.

p. 62    **stress stimulates tumor growth:** Sapolsky, R. M., Donnelly, T. M. 1985. "Vulnerability to Stress-Induced Tumor Growth Increases with Age in Rats: Role of Glucocorticoids." *Endocrinology.* 117(2):662–666.

Spiegel, D. 1999. "Embodying the Mind in Psychooncology Research." *Advances in Mind-Body Research.* 15:267–271.

p. 62    **see cancer as a challenge:** Folkman, S. 1999. "Thoughts About Psychological Factors, PNI, and Cancer." *Advances in Mind-Body Medicine.* 15:255–259.

Greer, S. 1999. "Mind-Body Research in Psychooncology." *Advances in Mind-Body Medicine.* 15: 236–244.

Greer, S., et al. 1990. "Psychological Response to Breast Cancer and 15-year Outcome." *Lancet.* 335:49–50.

p. 63    **shift the locus of control:** Watson, M., Greer, S., Pruyn, J., Van den Borne, B. 1990. "Locus of Control and Adjustment to Cancer." *Psychological Reports.* 66:39–48.

p. 63    **Herbert Benson, M.D. and his colleagues:** Benson, H., Klipper, M. Z. 1975. *The Relaxation Response.* New York: William Morrow and Company.

p. 64    **relaxation has impressive results for people with cancer:** Bridge, L. R., et al. 1988. "Relaxation and Imagery in the Treatment of Breast Cancer." *British Medical Journal,* 297:1169–72.

Lyles, J. N., et al. 1982. "Efficacy of Relaxation Training and Guided Imagery in Reducing the Aversiveness of Cancer Chemotherapy." *Journal of Consulting and Clinical Psychology.* 50(4):509–524.

Syrjala, K. L., et al. 1995 "Relaxation and Imagery and Cognitive-Behavioral Training Reduce Pain During Cancer Treatment: A Controlled Clinical Trial." *Pain*. 63:189–198.

Wallace, K. G., 1997. "Analysis of Recent Literature Concerning Relaxation and Imagery Interventions for Cancer Pain." *Cancer Nursing*. 20(2):79–87.

p. 67    **psychologist Jeanne Achterberg:** Information presented by Achterberg can be found in the 1998 CCC transcripts titled, "Imagery and Cancer Treatment," and in the 1999 CCC transcripts titled, "Covering CAM Therapies in the Journals" at www.cmbm.org.

Achterberg, J., et al. 1989. "Behavioral Strategies for the Reduction of Pain and Anxiety Associated with Orthopedic Trauma." *Biofeedback and Self-Regulation*. 14(2):101–114.

Achterberg, J. 1985. *Imagery in Healing: Shamanism and Modern Medicine*. Boston: New Science Library, Shambala, 188–189.

Achterberg, J., Lawlis, F. 1982. "Imagery and Health Intervention." *Topics in Clinical Nursing*. January, 55–60.

p. 67    **two basic kinds of imagery techniques:** ibid.

p. 70    **active imagery:** Simonton, O. C., et al. 1978. *Getting Well Again*. Los Angeles: J.P. Tracher.

p. 71    **relaxation and guided imagery:** Bridge, L. R., et al. 1988. "Relaxation and Imagery in the Treatment of Breast Cancer." *British Medical Journal*. 297:1169–72.

Lyles, J. N., et al. 1982. "Efficacy of Relaxation Training and Guided Imagery in Reducing the Aversiveness of Cancer Chemotherapy." *Journal of Consulting and Clinical Psychology*. 50(4):509–524.

Wallace, K. G. 1997. "Analysis of Recent Literature Concerning Relaxation and Imagery Interventions for Cancer Pain." *Cancer Nursing*. 20(2):79–87.

p. 71    **Achterberg's research studies with Ryder:** Achterberg, J., Ryder M. S. 1989. "Effect of Music-Assisted Imagery on Neutrophils and Lymphocytes." *Biofeedback and Self-Regulation*. 14(3): 247–257.

p. 72    **Bernauer Newton:** Newton, B. W. 1982–1983. "The Use of Hypnosis in the Treatment of Cancer Patients." *American Journal of Clinical Hypnosis*. 25(2–3):105–109.

p. 72    **reduce severe pain:** Spiegel, D. 1985. "The Use of Hypnosis in Controlling Cancer Pain." *CA: A Cancer Journal for Clinicians* 35(4):221–231.

p. 72    **decrease nausea and vomiting:** Feldman, C. S., Salzberg, H. C. 1990. "The Role of Imagery in the Hypnotic Treatment of Adverse Reactions to Cancer Therapy." the *Journal of the South Carolina Medical Association*. May:303–306.

Spiegel, D., Moore, R. 1997. "Imagery and Hypnosis in the Treatment of Cancer Patients." *Oncology*. 11(8):1179–1795.

p. 73    **Pennebaker and his colleagues:** Pennebaker, J. W., et al. 1990. "Accelerating the Coping Process." *Journal of Personality and Social Psychology*. 58(3):528–537.

Pennebaker, J. W. 1993. "Putting Stress into Words: Health, Linguistic, and Therapeutic Implications." *Behavioral Research and Therapy*. 31(6):539–548.

Pennebaker, J. W., Kiecolt-Glaser, J. K., Glaser, R. 1988. "Disclosure of Traumas and Immune Function: Health Implications for Psychotherapy." *Journal of Personality and Social Psychology*. 63:75–84.

p. 73    **patients with rheumatoid arthritis and asthma:** Smyth J. M., et al. 1999. "Effects of Writing About Stressful Experiences on Symptom Reduction in Patients with Asthma or Rheumatoid Arthritis." *Journal of the American Medical Association*. 281(14): 1304–1309.

p. 74    **improvement in mood:** LaFontaine, T. P., et al. 1992. "Aerobic Exercise and Mood." *Sports Medicine*. 13(3):160–170.

p. 74    **exercise is an integral part of comprehensive cancer care:** Block, K. 1997. "The Role of the Self in Healthy Cancer Survivorship from the Front Lines of Treating Cancer." *Advances*. 13(1):6–26.

Fiatarone, M. A., et al. 1988. "Endogenous Opioids and the Exercise-Induced Augmentation of Natural Killer Cell Activity." *Journal Laboratory Clinical Medicine*. 112(5):544–552.

Winningham, M.L., MacVicar M.G. 1988. "The Effect of Aerobic Exercise on Patient Reports of Nausea." *Oncol Nurs Forum*. 15(4):447–50.

Winningham M.L., et al. 1989. "Effect of Aerobic Exercise on Body Weight and Composition in Breast Cancer Patients." *Oncol. Nurs. Forum*. 16(5): 147–55.

Winningham M.L. 1994. "Exercise and Cancer" in *Exercise for Prevention and Treatment of Illness*, Goldberg and Eliot, 301–15.

## Chapter 4: Healing Connections

p. 79    **mortality rates are consistently higher among the unmarried: :** Berkman, L. F. & Syme, S. L. 1979. "Social Networks, Host Resistance and Mortality: A Nine-Year Follow-Up Study of Alameda County Residents." *American Journal of Epidemiology*. 109(2):186–204.

p. 79    **study of residents of Alameda county:** ibid.

p. 80    **work of Janice Kiecolt-Glaser:** Kiecolt-Glaser J.K., et al. 1985. "Stress and Immune Function in Humans." In Ader, Felten, and Cohen, *Psychoneuroimmonology,* 854.
Kiecolt-Glaser J.K., et al. 1992. "Acute Psychological Stressors and Short-Term Immune Changes: What, Why, for Whom, and to What Extent?
Pennebaker, J.W., & Kiecolt-Glaser, J.K. & Glaser, R. 1988. "Disclosure of Traumas and Immune Function: Health Implications for Psychotherapy." *Journal of Personality and Social Psychology.* 63:75–84.

p. 80    **Canadian epidemiologist Elizabeth Maunsell:** Maunsell E., et al. 1995. "Social Support and Survival Among Women With Breast Cancer." *Cancer.* 76:631–7.

p. 81    **studies that have been done:** Rowland, J., et al. 1987. "Psychosocial Factors Affecting Consent to a Breast Cancer Chemoprevention Program (Abstract)." *Proc. Twenty-Third Annu.Mtg. Am. Soc. Clin. Oncol.* 6:226.
Rowland, J.H. 1989. "Intrapersonal Coping." In Jimmie C. Holland and Julia H. Rowland, *Handbook of Psychooncology.* New York:Oxford, 25–42.
Rowland, J.H. "Intrapersonal Resources: Social Support." In ibid., 59

p. 82    **psychologist Lawrence LeShan:** LeShan, L. 1994. *Cancer as a Turning Point, Revised Edition.* New York: Penguin Group.
LeShan, L. 1991. "A New Question in Studying Psychosocial Interventions and Cancer." *Journal of Personality and Social Psychology.* 61:899–909.

p. 83    **Steve Dunn:** Information presented by Dunn can be found in the 1998 CCC transcripts titled, "Providing Good Information to People with Cancer" and in the 1999 CCC transcripts titled, "Complementary and Alternative Therapies: Separating the Wheat from the Chaff" at www.cmbm.org.
Dunn's Web site is www.cancerguide.org.

p. 84    **Internet sources you find:** Boodman, S. G. August 10, 1999. "Medical Web Sites Can Steer You Wrong." *Washington Post.* Health/7.
Brody, J. E. August 31, 1999. "The Health Hazards of Point-and-Click Medicine." *New York Times.* D1.
Martin, J.P. August 31, 1999. "A World of Support." *Washington Post.* Health 10.
Martin, J. P. August 31, 1999. "One Couple's Struggle Gives Rise to Breast Cancer Web Site." *Washington Post.* Health.

p. 84    **groups concerned with spirituality and prayer:** Brown-Saltzman, K. 1997. "Replenishing the Spirit by Meditative Prayer and Guided Imagery" *Seminars in Oncology Nursing.* 13(4):255–259.

Levin, J. S. 1994. "Investigating the Epidemiologic Effects of Religious Experience: Findings, Explanations, and Barriers." In: Levin, J. S., ed. *Religion in Aging and Health: Theoretical Foundations and Methodological Frontiers.* Thousand Oaks, A Sage Publications, 3–17.

Levin, J. S. "Religious Factors in Aging, Adjustment and Health: A Theoretical Overview." In W.M. Clements (Ed.), *Religion, Aging, and Health: A Global Perspective.* (pp.133–146). New York: Haworth.

Levin, J.S. & Vanderpool, H.Y. 1992. "Religious Factors in Physical Health and the Prevention of Illness." In K.I. Pargament, K.I. Maton, & R.E. Hess (Eds.), *Religion and Prevention in Mental Health: Research, Vision, and Action* (pp. 83–103). New York: Haworth.

p. 85    **the research Spiegel did:** Spiegel, D., et al. 1981. "Group Support for Patients with Metastatic Cancer." *Archives of General Psychiatry.* 38:527–533.

p. 86    **the landmark study:** Spiegel, D., et al. 1989. "Effect of Psychosocial Treatment on Survival of Patients with Metastatic Breast Cancer." *Lancet.* 2:888–891.

p. 86    **psychiatrist Fawzy Fawzy:** Fawzy, F., et al. 1993. "Malignant Melanoma: Effects of an Early Structured Psychiatric Intervention, Coping, and Affective State on Recurrence and Survival 6 Years Later." *Archives of General Psychiatry.* 50:681–689.

Fawzy, F., et al. Aug 1990. "A Structured Psychiatric Intervention for Cancer Patients: I. Changes over Time in Methods of Coping and Affective Disturbance." *Archives of General Psychiatry.* 47: 720–725.

Fawzy, F., et al. Aug 1990. "A Structured Psychiatric Intervention for Cancer Patients: II. Changes over Time in Immunological Measures." *Archives of General Psychiatry.* 47:729–735.

p. 86    **study by Jeanne Richardson:** Richardson, J. L., et al. 1990. "The Effect of Compliance with Treatment on Survival Among Patients with Hematologic Malignancies." *Journal of Clinical Oncology.* 14(4):1128–1135.

## Chapter 5: Diet and Nutrition

p. 91    **Richard Doll and Richard Peto:** Doll, R., Peto, R., 1981. *The Causes of Cancer: Quantitative Estimates of the Avoidable Risks of Cancer in the United States Today.* New York: Oxford University Press.

p. 92    **contaminants in food:** Information on contaminants in food presented by Dr. Davis can be found in the 1999 CCC transcripts titled, "Addressing the Environmental Causes of Cancer" at www.cmbm.org.
The World Resources Institute Web site is www.wri.org.
Bradlaw, H. L., et al. 1995. "Effects of Pesticides on the Ration of 16 Alpha/2-Hydraxyestrone: A Biologic Marker of Breast Cancer Risk." *Environmental Health Perspectives.* 103(Suppl 7):147–150.

p. 93    **whole grains:** Jacobs, D. R., Jr., Marquart, L., et al. 1998. "Whole Grain Intake and Cancer: An Expanded Review and Meta-Analysis." *Nutrition and Cancer.* 30(2):85–96.

p. 93    **cruciferous vegetables:** Fahey, J. W., et al. 1997. "Broccoli Sprouts: An Exceptionally Rich Source of Inducers of Enzymes that Protect Against Chemical Carcinogens." *Proceedings National Academy of Science.* 94(19):10367–10372.
Kali, M. A., et al. 1996. "Effects of Dietary Broccoli on Human In Vivo Drug Metabolizing Enzymes: Evaluation of Caffeine, Estrone and Chlorzoxazone Metabolism." 17(4):793–799.
Nestle, M. 1997. "Broccoli Sprouts in Cancer Prevention." *Nutrition Reviews.* 56(4):127–130.
Walaszek, Z., et al. 1986. "Dietary Glucarate As Anti-Promoter of 7,12-dimethylbenz[a]antracene-induced Mammary Tumorigenesis." *Carcinogenesis.* 7(9):1463–1466.
Walaszek, Z. 1990. "Research Update: AICR Study Find Vegetable Compound Effective Against Cancer." *A.I.C.R. Newsletter.* 27:12.

p. 93    **soy:** Arnot, R. *The Breast Cancer Prevention Diet.* Boston: Little Brown & Co.
Burros, M. January 26, 2000. "Doubts Cloud Rosy News on Soy." *New York Times.* D1.
Cline, J. M., Hughes, C. L. 1998. "Phytochemicals for the Prevention of Breast and Endometrial Cancer." *Cancer Treatment Resviews.* 94:107–134.
Katdore, M., et al. 1998. "Inhibition of Aberrant Proliferation and Induction of Apoptosis in Pre-Neoplastic Human Mammary Epithelial Cells by Natural Phytochemicals." *Oncol Rep.* Mar; 5(2):311–315.
Kurzer, M. S., Xu, X, 1997. "Dietary Phytoestrogens." *Annual. Review Nutrition.* 17:353–381.
McMichael-Phillips, D. F., et al. 1998. "Effects of Soy-Protein Supplementation on Epithelial Proliferation in the Histologically Normal Human Breast." *American Journal of Clinical Nutrition.* 68(6Suppl):1431S–1435S.

Zava, D. T., Duwe, G. 1997. "Estrogenic and Antiproliferative Properties of Genistein and Other Flavonoids in Human Breast Cancer Cells In Vitro." *Nutrition and Cancer.* 27(1)31–40.

Zhou, Y., Lee, A. S. 1998. "Mechanism for the Suppression of the Mammalian Stress Response by Genistein, an Anticancer Phytoestrogen from Soy." *Journal of the National Cancer Institute* 90(5):381–388.

p. 93    **antioxidant vitamins:** Omenn, G. S. 1996. "Micronutrients (Vitamins and Minerals) As Cancer-Preventive Agents." *IARC Scientific Publications.* 139:33–45.

Prasad, K. N., Kumar, A., et al. 1999. "High Doses of Multiple Antioxidant Vitamins: Essential Ingredients in Improving the Efficacy of Standard Cancer Therapy." *Journal of the American College of Nutrition.* 18(1):13–25.

Prasad, K. N., Cole, W., Hovland, P. 1998. "Cancer Prevention Studies: Past, Present, and Future Directions." *Nutrition.* 14:(197–210).

p. 96    **"mind-body skills" group:** Information on mind-body skills groups can be found in the 1999 CCC transcripts, titled "Mind-Body Skills Groups for Cancer" at www.cmbm.org.

p. 96    **"mindfulness" meditation:** Hanh, T N. 1991. *Peace Is Every Step.* New York: Bantam Books.

p. 97    **Dr. Jeffrey Bland:** Information presented by Dr. Bland can be found in the 1999 CCC transcripts titled, "Nutritional Guidelines for People with Cancer" at www.cmbm.org.

Bland, J. 1998. "The Use of Complementary Medicine for Healthy Aging." *Alternative Therapies.* 4(4):42–48.

Bland, J., Levin, B. 1997. "Nutritional Support for a Biopsychological Approach to Cancer Therapy." *Advances: The Journal of Mind-Body Health.* 13(1)26–29.

Bland, J., Bralley, J. A. 1992. "Nutritional Upregulation of Hepatic Detoxication Enzymes." *Journal of Applied Nutrition.* 44(3–4):1–18.

Goodwin, J. S. & Tangum, M. R. 1998. "Battline Quackery: Attitudes About Micronutrient Suppliments in American Academic Medicine" 158(20):2187–2191.

p. 97    **phytochemicals:** A.I.C.R. 1995. "Phytochemicals for Cancer Protection." *A.I.C.R. Newsletter.* Winter(46):11.

Katdore, M., et al. 1998. "Inhibition of Aberrant Proliferation and Induction of Apoptosis in Pre-Neoplastic Human Mammary Epithelial Cells by Natural Phytochemicals." *Oncololgy Report* 5(2)311–315.

p. 98    **free radicals:** Harman, D. "Free Radical Theory of Aging: Role of Free Radicals in the Origination and Evolution of Life, Aging, and Disease Processes" In John E. Johnson, Jr., et al., eds., *Free Radicals, Aging, and Degenerative Diseases.* New York: Alan R. Liss.
Weijl, N. I., et al. 1997. "Free Radicals and Antioxidants in Chemotherapy-Induced Toxicity." *Cancer Treatment Reviews.* 23:209–40.

p. 98    **vitamin A, C, E:** Gey, F. K. 1998. "Vitamins E plus C and Inter-acting Conutrients Required for Optimal Health." *Biofactors.* 113–74.
Sankaranarayanan, R., Mathew, B. 1996. "Retinoids as Cancer-Preventive Agents." *IARC Scientific Publications.* 139:47–59.
1998. "Antioxidants: Vitamin E May Cut Prostate Cancer Risk." *Harvard Health Letter.* 23(7):7.
Zhang, S., et al. 1999. "Dietary Carotenoids and Vitamins A, C, and E and Risk of Breast Cancer." *Journal of the National Cancer Institute.* 91(6):547–556.

p. 98    **Beta-Carotene:** Jumaan, AO, et al. 1999. "Beta-Carotene Intake and Risk of Postmenopausal Breast Cancer." *Epidemiology.* 10(1):49–53.
Pool-Zobel, B. L., et al. 1997. "Consumption of Vegetables Reduces Genetic Damage in Humans: First Results of a Human Intervention Trial with Carotenoid-Rich Foods." *Carcinogenesis.* 18(9):1847–1850.
Rock, C. L. 1997. "Caroteniods: Biology and Treatment." *Pharmacology Therapeutics.* 75(3):185–197.
Zeigler, R. G. 1991. "Vegetables, Fruits, and Carotenoids and the Risk of Cancer." *American Journal of Clinical Nutrition.* 53 (Suppl.):251S–259S.

p. 98    **selenium:** Dorgan, J. F., et al. 1998. "Relationship of Serum Carotenoids, Retinol, Alpha-Tocopheraol, and Selenium with Breast Cancer Risk: Results from a Prospective Study in Columbia, Missouri." *Cancer Causes and Control.*
Schaffer, E. M., Liu, J. Z., Milner, J. A. 1996. "Inhibition of 7,12-dimethylbenz(a)anthracene (DMBA)-Induced Mammary DNA Adducts by Dietary Supplementation with Selenium and Garlic Constitutents(meeting abstract)." *Proceedings of the Annual Meeting of the American Association of Cancer Research.* 37:A1924

p. 98    **bioflavinoids:** Elangovan, V., Sekar, N., Govindasamy, S. 1994. "Chemopreventive Potential of Dietary Bioflavonoids Against 20-Methylcholanthrene-induced Tumorigenesis." *Cancer Letter.* 87:107–113.

Kuo, S. M. 1997. "Dietary Flavonoid and Cancer Prevention: Evidence and Potential Mechanism." *Critical Reviews in Oncogenesis.* 8(1):47–69.

p. 98    **grapes:** Jang, M., Cai, L., Udeani, G. O., et al. 1997. "Cancer Chemopreventive Activity of Resveratrol, a Natural Product Derived from Grapes." *Science.* 275:(218–220).

Mgbonywbi, O. P., Russo, J., Russo, I. H. 1998. "Anitproliferative Effect of Resveratrol on Human Breast Epithelial Cells." *International Journal of Oncology.* 12(4):865–869.

p. 98    **tea:** Nagata, C., et al. 1998. "Association of Coffee, Green Tea, and Caffeine Intakes with Serum Concentration of Estradiol and Sex Hormone-Binding Globulin in Premenopausal Japanese Women." *Nutrition and Cancer.* 30(1)21–24.

Nakachi, K., et al. 1998. "Influence of Drinking Green Tea on Breast Cancer Malignancy among Japanese Patients." *Japanese Journal of Cancer Research.* 89(3):254–261.

Sadzuka, Y., et al. 1998. "Modulation of Cancer Chemotherapy by Green Tea." *Clinical Cancer Research.* 4(1):153–6.

p. 98    **"limonene":** Crowell, P. L., Gould, M. N. 1994. "Chemoprevention and Therapy of Cancer by *d*-limonene." *Critical Reviews on Oncology.* 5:1–22.

Gould, M. N. 1995. "Prevention and Therapy of Mammary Cancer by Monoterpenes." *Journal of Cellular Biochemistry.* 22(Suppl):139–144.

Gould, M. N. 1997. "Cancer Chemoprevention and Therapy by Monoterpenes." *Environmental Health Perspectives.* 105(Suppl 4):977–979.

p. 98    **soy products can reduce the overstimulation:** Information on soy presented by Dr. Bland can be found in the 1999 CCC transcripts titled, "Nutritional Guidelines for People with Cancer" at www.cmbm.org.

p. 99    **Omega-6:** Cameron, E., Bland, J., Marcuson, R. 1989. "Divergent Effects of Omega-6 and Omega-3 Fatty Acids on Mammary Tumor Development in C3H/Heston Mice Treated with DMBA." *Nutrition Research.* 9:383–393.

Simonsen, V., van't Veer, P., et al. 1998. "Adipose Tissue Omega-3 and Omega-6 Fatty Acid Content and Breast Cancer in the EURAMIC Study." *American Journal of Epidemiology.* 147(4):342–352.

p. 99    **high fat diets decrease immune function:** Malter, M., et al. 1989. "Natural Killer Cells, Vitamins and Other Blood Components of Vegetarian and Omnivorous Men." *Nutrition and Cancer.* 12:271–278.

Fong, A., et al. 1990. "Mechanisms of Anti-Carcinogenesis by Indole-3-Carbinol:Studies of Enzyme Induction, Electrophile-Scavenging, and Inhibition of Alfatoxin B1 Activation. *Biochemical Pharmacology.* 39:19–26.

p. 99    **animal fats increase the amount of PGE:** Bland, J. 1996. "Phytonutrition, Phytotherapy, and Phytopharmacology." *Alternative Therapies.* 2(6):73–76.

Broitman S. A., Cannizzo, Jr., F., 1992. "A Model System for Studying Nutritional Interventions on Colon Tumor Growth: Effects of Marine Oil." In M. M. Jacobs, ed. *Exercise, Calories, Fat and Cancer.* New York: Plenum Press.

p. 100    **bioavailability of sex hormones:** Adlercreutz, H. 1991. "Diet and Sex Hormone Metabolism." In Rowland, I.R., et al., *Nutrition, Toxicity and Cancer.* Florida: CRC Press, 137–195.

p. 100    **flaxseeds:** Adlercreutz, H., Fotsis, T. Heikkinen R., et al. 1982. "Excretion of the Lignans Enterolactone and Enterodiol and of Equol in Omnivorous and Vegetarian Postmenopausal Women and in Women with Breast Cancer." *Lancet.* Ii:1295–1299.

Thompson, I. U., Rickard, S. E., et al. 1996. "Flaxseed and Its Lignan and Oil Components Reduce Mammary Tumor Growth." *Carcinogenesis.* 17(6):1373–6.

Thompson, l.U., Siedl, M. M., et al. 1996. "Antituomorigenic Effect of a Mammalian Lignan Precursor from Flaxseed." *Nutriton and Cancer.* 26(2):159–165.

p. 100    **Omega-3 fatty acids:** Fernandes, G., Venkatraman, J. T. 1993. "Role of Omega-3 Fatty Acids in Health and Disease." *Nutritional Research.* 13:S19-S45.

Glaspa, J., Bagga, D. 1998. "Re: Dietary Modulation of Omega-3/Omega-6 Polyunsaturated Fatty Acid Ratios in Patients with Breast Cancer." *Journal of the National Cancer Institute.* 90(8):629–631.

Gogos, C. A., Ginopoulos, P., et al. 1998. "Dietary Omega-3 Polyunsaturated Fatty Acids Plus Vitamin E Restore Immunodeficiency and Prolong Survival for Severely Ill Patients with Generalized Malignancy: A Randomized Control Trial." *Cancer.* 82(2):395–402.

Imoberdorf, R. 1997. "Immuno-Nutrition: Designer Diets in Cancer." *Supportive Care in Cancer.* 5(5):381–386.

Simonsen, V., van't Veer, P., et al. 1998. "Adipose Tissue Omega-3 and Omega-6 Fatty Acid Content and Breast Cancer in the EURAMIC Study." *American Journal of Epidemiology* 147(4):342–352.

p. 101    fish: Favero, A., ct al. 1998. "Diet and Risk of Breast Cancer: Major Findings from an Italian Case-Control Study." *Biomedicine and Pharmacotherapy.* 52(3):109–115.

Kaizer, L., Boyd, N. F., et al. 1989. "Fish Consumption and Breast Cancer Risk: An Ecological Study. " *Nutrition and Cancer.* 12:61–68.

Kune, G. A. 1990. "Eating Fish Protects Against Some Cancers: Epidemiological and Experimental Evidence for a Hypothesis." *Journal of Nutrional Medicine.* 1:139–144.

Lund, E., et al. 1990. "Reduced Breast Cancer Mortality Among Fishermen's Wives in Norway." *Cancer Causes and Control.* 4:283–287.

p. 101    **Dietary sugar has been shown:** Information on sugars presented by Dr. Bland can be found in the 1999 CCC transcripts titled, "Nutritional Guidelines for People with Cancer" at www.cmbm.org.

p. 101    **Strawberries and blueberries:** Information on strawberries and blueberries presented by Dr. Daniel Nixon can be found in the 1999 CCC transcripts titled, "Nutritional Guidelines for People with Cancer" at www.cmbm.org.

Nixon, D. W. 1994. *The Cancer Recovery Eating Plan: The Right Foods to Help Fuel Your Recovery.* New York: Times Books.

p. 102    **fiber also promotes the excretion of hormones:** Adlercreutz, H. "Diet and Sex Hormone Metabolism." In Rowland, I. R., et al., *Nutrition, Toxicity and Cancer.* Florida: CRC Press, 137–195.

Goldin, B., et al. 1982. "Estrogen Excretion Patterns and Plasma Levels in Vegetarian and Omnivorous Women." *New England Journal of Medicine.* 307925):1542–6.

Goldin, B. R., Adlercreutz, H., et al. 1981. "Effect of Diet on Excretion of Estrogens in Pre-and Post Menopausal Women. *Cancer Research.* 41(9 Pt 2):3771–3773.

p. 102    **fiber lowers cancer risk:** Adlercreutz, H., Hamalainen, E., Gorbach, S. L., et al. 1989. "Diet and Plasma Androgens in Postmenopausal Vegetarian and Omnivorous Women and Postmenopausal Women with Breast Cancer." *American Journal of Clinical Nutrition.* 49:433–442.

Kritchevsky, D. 1997. "Dietary Fibre and Cancer." *European Journal of Cancer Prevention.* 6:435–441.

Stoll, B. A. 1997. "Macronutrient Supplements May Reduce Breast Cancer Risk: How, When, and Which? *European Journal of Clinical Nutrition.* 51(9):573–577.

p. 103    **"Paleolithic diet":** Eaton, S. B., Konner, M. 1985. "Paleolithic Nutrition: A Consideration of Its Nature and Current Implications." *New England Journal of Medicine.* 312(5):283–289.

p. 104    **Dr. Daniel Nixon:** Information presented by Dr. Nixon can be found in the 1999 CCC transcripts titled, "Nutritional Guidelines for People with Cancer" and "Colon Cancer" at www.cmbm.org.

p. 105    **Finnish ATBC trial:** Heinonen, O. P., Albanes, D. 1994. "Alpha-Tococopherol, Beta-Carotene Cancer Prevention Study Group." *New England Journal of Medicine.* 339:1029–1035.

p. 105    **NCI CARET:** Omenn, G. S., Goodman, G. E., Thornquist, M. D., et al. 1996. "Effects of a Combination of Beta-Carotene and Vitamin A on Lung Cancer and Cardiovascular Disease." *New England Journal of Medicine.* 334:1150–1155.

p. 106    **Garlic:** Abdullah, T. H., et al. 1989. "Enhancement of Natural Killer Cell Activity in AIDS with Garlic." *Deutsche Zeitschrift fur Onkologie.* 24:52–53.
A.I.C.R. 1995. "Phytochemicals for Cancer Protection." *AICR. Newsletter.* Winter(46):11.
Lau, B.H.S. 1991. "Garlic Compounds Modulate Macrophage and T-Lymphocyte Functions." *Molecular Biotherapy.* 3:103–107.

p. 106    **antioxidants:** see antioxidant vitamins above.

p. 107    **lycopene antioxidant:** Giovannucci, E., Clinton, S. K. 1998. "Tomatoes, Lycopene, and Prostate Cancer." *Prostate Cancer.* pp. 129–139. The Arthur G. James Cancer Hospital and Research Institute. The Ohio State University.
Stahl, W., Sies, H. 1992. "Uptake of Lycopene and Its Geometrical Isomers Is Greater from Heat-Processed Than from Unprocessed Tomato Juice in Humans." *Journal of Nutrition.* 122:2161–2166.

## Chapter 6: *Traditional Chinese Medicine*

p. 109    **James Reston:** Reston, J. "Now, About My Operation in Peking." *New York Times.* July 26, 1971, 1.

p. 110    **the world of traditional chinese medicine (TCM):** Some of the many available books on TCM are listed in our bibliography.

p. 117    **Dr. Ming Tian:** Information presented by Dr. Tian can be found in the 1998 CCC transcripts titled, "The Uses of Chinese Medicine" and in the 1999 CCC transcripts titled, "Chinese Medicine and Herbal Therapies" at www.cmbm.org.

p. 117 **"Consensus Conference":** Acupuncture. 1997. *NIH Consensus Statement.* 15(5):1–34.

p. 120 **herbs:** ibid.

Beinfield, H., Korngold, E. 1991. *Between Heaven and Earth: A Guide to Chinese Medicine.* New York: Ballantine.

Boik, J. 1995. *Cancer &Natural Medicine: A Textbook of Basic Science and Clinical Research.* Princeton, MN: Oregon Medical. 1995.

p. 121 *Panax ginseng:* Xiaoguang, C., et al. 1998. "Cancer Chemopreventive and Therapeutic Activities of Red Ginseng." *Journal of Ethnopharmacology.* 60(1):71–78.

Cheng, X. J., et al. 1986. "Comparison of Action of Panax Ginsenosides and Panax Quinquonosides on Anti-Warm Stress in Mice." *Journal of Shenyang College of Pharmacy.* 3(3):170–172.

p. 121 **group of 188 patients with advanced nasopharyngeal cancer:** Xu, G. Z., et al. 1989. "Chinese Herb 'Destagnation' Series I: Combination of Radiation with Destagnation in the Treatment of Nasopharyngeal Carcinoma (NPC): A Prospective Randomized Trial on 188 Cases." *International Journal of Radiation Oncology, Biology and Physics.* 16(2):297–300.

p. 121 **traditional herbal combination:** Ling, H. Y. 1989. "Preliminary Study of Traditional Chinese Medicine-Western Medicine Treatment of Patients with Primary Liver Carcinoma." *Chung HhisI Chieh Ho Tsa Chih (Chinese Journal of Modern Developments in Traditional Medicine).* 9(6):325, 348–349.

p. 121 **study of 285 people:** Hong-Yen Hsu. 1982. *Treating Cancer with Chinese Herbs.* Long Beach, CA: Oriental Healing Arts Institute.

p. 122 **Dr. Yan Su's work:** Information presented by Dr. Yan Su can be found in the 1998 CCC transcripts titled, "The Uses of Chinese Medicine" at www.cmbm.org.

p. 122 **Dr. Alexander Sun:** Sun, A. S., et al. 1999. "Phase I/II Study of Stage III and IV Non-Small Cell Lung Cancer Patients Taking a Specific Dietary Supplement." *Nutrition and Cancer.* 34 (1):62–69.

Sun, A.S., et al. 1999. "Nutritional Support for NSCLC Patients." *Food Therapy.* Information presented by Dr. Sun can be found in the 1999 CCC transcripts titled, "Chinese Medicine and Herbal Therapies" at www.cmbm.org.

p. 125 **study from the First Medical College:** Zhou, L., et al. First Medical College of PLA, Guangzhou, China. "Mechanisms of the Anti-Tumor Effect of QiGong Waiqi (emitted qi). 3rd National Academic Conference on Qi Gong Science. 88Eb:1990.

p. 127　**Dr. Chen's well-researched PC-SPES:** Information presented by Dr. Chen can be found in the 1999 CCC transcripts titled, "Chinese Medicine and Herbal Therapies" at www.cmbm.org. See Chapter 9

## Chapter 7: Immunomodulating Substances: Coley's Toxin, Mistletoe, MTH–68

p. 130　**resources on the history of medicine include:** Ackerknecht, E. A. 1982. *A Short History of Medicine,* rev. ed. Baltimore: Johns Hopkins University Press.
Lyons, A. and Petrocelli, R. J. *Medicine: An Illustrated History.* New York: Abradale Press. Harry Abrams: 1987.

p. 130　**Sir Macfarlane Burnet:** Burnet, M. 1957. "Cancer—A Biological Approach." *British Medical Journal.* I:779–786.
Burnet, M. 1971. *Genes, Dreams, and Realities.* Aylesbury: Medical Technical Publishing.

p. 135　**DeVita's text:** DeVita, V.T., et al. 1992. *Cancer: Principles of Oncology.* J.B. Lippincott Co.

p. 135　**Dr. Ralph Kleef:** Information presented by Dr. Kleef can be found in the 1998 CCC transcripts titled, "Immunotherapies" at www.cmbm.org.

p. 136　**Dr. Alan Freeman:** Information presented by Dr. Freeman can be found in the 1998 CCC transcripts titled, "Immunotherapies" at www.cmbm.org.

p. 136　**Dr. Tibor Bakacs:** Information presented by Dr. Bakacs can be found in the 1998 CCC transcripts titled, "New Biological Therapies" at www.cmbm.org.

p. 138　**Dr. Josef Beuth:** Information presented by Dr. Beuth can be found in the 1998 CCC transcripts titled, "Issues in Research on Complementary and Alternative Cancer Treatments" and "Immunotherapies" at www.cmbm.org.

p. 139　**Rudolf Steiner:** Information on Rudolf Steiner can be found in the 1999 CCC transcripts titled, "Anthroposophical Medicine" at www.cmbm.org.

p. 139　**mistletoe:** Information on mistletoe presented by Dr. Beuth can be found in the 1998 CCC transcripts titled, "Issues in Research on Complementary and Alternative Cancer Treatments" and "Immunotherapies" at www.cmbm.org.
Gorter, R. W. 1998. *Iscador:Mistletoe Preperations Used in Anthroposophically Extended Cancer Treatment.* Basel, Switzerland: Verlag fur GanzheitsMedizin.

## Chapter 8: Nature's Pharmacy:
## Phytonutrients and Nutraceuticals

p. 145    **Dr. Judah Folkman:** Folkman, J. 1976. "The Vascularization of Tumors." *Scientific American.* 234:58–64.

p. 145    **bovine (calf) cartilage:** Prudden, J. 1985. "The Treatment of Human Cancer with Agents Prepared from Bovine Cartilage." *Journal of Biology R. M.* 590–5.

p. 145    **research on shark cartilage:** Haney, D. Q. 1998. "Shark Cartilage Nixed Vs. Tumors." *Associated Press.* October 30.

p. 146    **Charles Simone, M.D.:** Information presented by Dr. Simone can be found in the 1998 CCC transcripts titled, "New Biological Therapies" at www.cmbm.org.

p. 148    **Essiac Tea:** Information on Essaic tea can be found in the 1998 CCC transcripts titled, "Herbal Therapies" at www.cmbm.org.

p. 149    **Hoxsey's formula:** ibid.

p. 149    **Dr. James Duke:** ibid.
Duke, J., Foster, S. 1990. *Peterson's Field Guide to Medicinal Plants.* Boston: Houghton-Mifflin.

p. 149    *Maitake-D:* Nanba, H. 1995. "Results of Non-Controlled Clinical Study for Various Cancer Patients Using Maitake D-Fraction." *Explore.* 6(5):19–21.

p. 150    **Dr. Cun Zhaung:** Information presented by Dr. Cun can be found in the 1998 CCC transcripts titled, "New Biological Therapies" at www.cmbm.org.

p. 151    **Green tea, with reports of chemoprevention:** Kaegi, E. 1998. "Unconventional Therapies for Cancer: 2. Green Tea. The Task Force on Alternative Therapies of the Canadian Breast Cancer Research Initiative." *Canadian Medical Association Journal.* 158(8):1033–1035.
Katiyar, S.K., et al. 1997. "Tea Antioxidants in Cancer Chemoprevention." *Journal of Cellular Biochemistry.* 27(Suppl):59–67.
Komori, A., et al. 1993. "Anticarcinogenic Activity of Green Tea Polyphenols." *Japanese Journal of Clinical Oncology.* 23:186–190.

p. 152    **Dr. Richard Willis:** Information presented by Dr. Willis can be found in the 1998 CCC transcripts titled, "New Therapies for Breast Cancer" at www.cmbm.org.

p. 153    **Melatonin:** ibid.

p. 154    **inhibitory effect on estrogen-responsive cells:** ibid.

p. 154    **immune response and melatonin:** Lissoni, P., et al. 1993. "Neuroimmunotherapy of Advanced Solid Neoplasms with Single Evening Subcutaneous Injection of Low-dose Interleukin and Melatonin." *European Journal of Cancer.* 29A(2):185–189.

Lissoni, P., et al. 1993. "A Study of the Mechanisms Involved in the Immunostimulatory Action of the Pineal Hormone in Cancer Patients." *Oncology*. 50(6):399–400.

Lissoni, P., et al. 1994. "Efficacy of the Concomitant Administration of the Pineal Hormone Melatonin in Cancer Immunotherapy with Low-dose IL-2 in Patients with Advanced Solid Tumors Who Had Progressed on IL-2 Alone." *Oncology*. 51(4):344–347.

Lissoni, P., et al. 1994. "Pineal-opioid System Interactions in the Control of Immunoinflammatory Responses." *Annals of the New York Academy of Sci*ence. 741:191–196.

p. 154    **study by Dr. Ann Massion:** Massion, A. O., et al. 1995. "Meditation, Melatonin and Breast/Prostate Cancer: Hypothesis and Preliminary Data." *Medical Hypotheses*. 44:39–46.

p. 154    **David Blask, Ph.D.:** Information presented by Dr. Blask can be found in the 1998 CCC transcripts titled, "New Therapies for Breast Cancer" at www.cmbm.org.

p. 155    **cancer metastatic to the brain:** Lissoni, P., et al. 1994. "A Randomized Study with the Pineal Hormone Melatonin Versus Supportive Care Alone in Patients with Brain Metastases Due to Solid Neoplasms." *Cancer*. 73:699–701.

Lissoni, P., et al. 1991. "Clinical Results with the Pineal Hormone Melatonin in Advanced Cancer Resistant to Standard Antitumor Therapies." *Oncology*. 48(6):448–450.

Lissoni, P., et al. 1992. "Randomized Study with Pineal Hormone Melatonin vs. Supportive Care Alone in Advanced Nonsmall Cell Lung Cancer Resistant to Firstline Chemotherapy Containing Cisplatin." *Oncology*. 49(5):336–339.

Lissoni, P., et al. 1992. "Biological and Clinical Results of a Neuroimmunotherapy with Interleukin-2 and the Pineal Hormone Melatonin as a First Line Treatment in Advanced Nonsmall Cell Lung Cancer." *British Journal of Cancer*. 66(1):155–158.

## Chapter 9: Prostate and Breast Cancers

p. 163    **AUA guidelines:** Middleton, Richard G., et al. 1995. "Prostate Cancer Clinical Guidelines Panel Summary Report on the Management of Clinically Localized Prostate Cancer." *Journal of Urology*. 154: 2144–2148.

p. 163    **report in *Oncology*:** Litwin, Mark S., et al. 1995. "Quality-of-Life Outcomes in Men Treated for Localized Prostate Cancer." *Journal of the American Medical Association*. 273(2):129–135.

p. 163    **making decisions on incomplete data:** Morra, M., Potts, E. 1994. *Choices,* revised ed. New York: Avon Books.

p. 164    **Dr. Robert Atkins:** Information presented by Dr. Atkins can be found in the 1998 CCC transcripts titled, "New Therapies for Prostate Cancer" and "The Dietary Treatment of Cancer (Part I)" and in the 1999 CCC transcripts titled, "Providing Integrative Care III" at www.cmbm.org.

Atkins, R. C. 1999. *Dr. Atkins' New Diet Revolution: Revised and Updated.* New York: Avon Books, Inc.

p. 165    **Dr. William Fair:** Information presented by Dr. Fair can be found in the 1998 CCC transcripts titled, "New Therapies for Prostate Cancer" and in the 1999 CCC transcripts titled, "Colon Cancer" at www.cmbm.org.

p. 166    **Dr. Sophie Chen:** Information presented by Dr. Chen can be found in the 1998 CCC transcripts titled, "New Therapies for Prostate Cancer" and in the 1999 CCC transcripts titled, "Chinese Medicine and Herbal Therapies" at www.cmbm.org.

Chen, S., et al. 1997. "Regulation of androgen receptor (AR) and PSA expression in androgen-responsive human prostate LNCaP cells by ethanolic extracts of the Chinese herbal preparation PC-SPES." *Biochemistry and Molecular Biology International.* 42(3):535–44.

Halicka, H.D., Chen, S., et al. 1997. "Apoptosis and Cell Cycle Effects Induced by Extracts of Chinese Herbal Preperation PC-SPES." *International Journal of Oncology.* 11:437–448.

Hsieh, T., et al. 1997. "Regulation of Androgen Receptor (AR) and Prostate Specific Antigen (PSA) Expression in the Androgen-Responsive Human Prostate LNCaP Cells by Ethanolic Extracts of the Chinese Herbal Preparation, PC-SPES." *Biochem. Mol. Biol. Int.* 42(3):535–44.

p. 166    **saw palmetto:** Champpault, G., Patel, J.D., and Bonnard, A.M. 1984. "A Double-Blind Trial of an Extract of the Plant *Serenoa repens* in Benign Prostatic Hyperplasia." *British Journal of Clinical Pharmacology.* 18(3):461–462.

p. 167    **article in the *New England Journal of Medicine*:** DiPaola, R. S., et al. 1998. "Clinical and Biologic Activity of an Estrogenic Herbal Combination (PC-SPES) in Prostate Cancer." *N. E. J. M.* 339(12):785–91.

p. 168    **Dr. Richard Rivlin:** Information presented by Dr. Rivlin can be found in the 1998 CCC transcripts titled "New Therapies for Prostate Cancer" at www.cmbm.org.

p. 171    **risk factors for breast cancer:** Herbert, J. R. & Rosen, A. 1996. "Nutritional, Socioeconomic, and Reproductive Factors in Relation to Female Breast Cancer Mortality: Findings from a Cross-national Study." *Cancer Detect. Prevent.* 20:234–44.

p. 172    **connections between diet, and breast cancer:** Evans, W. G. 1995. "Effects of Exercise on Body Composition and Functional Capacity of the Elderly." *J. Geront. A. Bio. Sci. Med. Sci.* 50 Spec No:147.

Favero, A., et al. 1998. "Diet and Risk of Breast Cancer: Major Findings from an Italian Case-Control Study." *Biomed. Pharmacother.* 52(3):109–15.

Goard, M., et al. 1995. "Dietary Fat and the Risk of Breast Cancer: a Prospective Study of 25,892 Norwegian Women." *Int. J. Cancer.* 63:13.

Howe, G. R., et al. 1990. "Dietary Factor and Risk of Breast Cancer: Combined Analysis of 12 Case-Control Studies." *J. Natl. Cancer.* 82:561–9.

Ingram, D. M., et al. 1991. "The Role of Diet in the Development of Breast Cancer: A Case-Control Study of Patients with Breast Cancer, Benign Epithelial Hyperplasia and Fibrocystic Disease of the Breast." *British Journal of Cancer.* 64:187–191.

Herbert, J. R., et al. 1998. "The Effect of Dietary Exposures on Recurrence and Mortality in Early Stage Breast Cancer." *Breast Cancer Research Treatment* 51(1):17–28.

Toniolo, P., et al. 1989. "Calorie-providing Nutrients and Risk of Breast Cancer." *Journal of the National Cancer Institute.* 81(4):278–286.

Toniolo, P., et al. 1994. "Consumption of Meat, Animal Products, Protein, and Fat and Risk of Breast Cancer: A Prospective Cohort Study in New York." *Epidemiology.* 5:391.

p. 172    **Dr. Devra Davis, Ph.D.:** Information presented by Dr. Davis can be found in the 1999 CCC transcripts titled, "Strategies for Prevention" at www.cmbm.org.

p. 174    **rats fed miso:** Hiryama, T. 1982. "Relationship of Soybean Paste Soup Intake to Gastric Cancer." *Nutrition and Cancer.* 3:223–233.

p. 174    **induces apoptosis:** Katdore, M., et al. 1998. "Inhibition of Aberrant Proliferation and Induction of Apoptosis in Pre-Neoplastic Human Mammary Epithelial Cells by Natural Phytochemicals." *Oncol. Rep.* 5(2)311–315.

Zhou, Y, Lee, A. S. 1998. "Mechanism for the Suppression of the Mammalian Stress Response by Genistein, an Anticancer Phytoestrogen from Soy." *Journal of the National Cancer Institute.* 90(5):381–388.

p. 174    **inhibits angiogenesis, induces differentiation:** Kurzer, M. S., Xu, X. 1997. "Dietary Phytoestrogens." *Annual Review of Nutrition* 17:353–381.

p. 175    **Dr. Charles Simone:** Information presented by Dr. Simone can be found in the 1998 CCC transcripts titled, "New Biological Therapies" at www.cmbm.org.

## Chapter 10: Therapeutic Diets

p. 178    **Max B. Gerson:** Ward, P .S. June 1988. "History of Gerson Therapy" contract report for the U.S. Congress Office of Technology Assessment.

p. 179    **essential elements in his regimen:** Hildenbrand, G. March-June 1987. "Let's Set the Record Straight, Part 5–Bread, Propaganda, and Circuses." *The Healing Newsletter*
Gerson, M. 1978. "The Cure of Advanced Cancer by Diet Therapy: A Summary of 30 Years of Clinical Experimentation." *Physiological Chemistry and Physics.* 10:4499–4464. Cited in U.S. Congress Office of Technology Assessment. 1990. "Unconventional Cancer Treatments." Washington D. C.: Government Printing Office, 45.

p. 180    **in 1949, he reported:** Gerson, M. 1949. "Effects of a Combined Dietary Regime on Patients with Malignant Tumors." *Experimental Medicine and Surgery.* 7(4)299–317.

p. 180    **rewrote *A Cancer Therapy:*** Gerson, M. *A Cancer Therapy:Results of Fifty Cases.* Del Mar, CA: Totality Books, 1977.

p. 180    **Dr. Peter Lechner:** Lechner, P. 1987. "The Role of a Modified Gerson Therapy in the Treatment of Cancer." Typescript, Second Department of Surgery, Landeskranhenhaus, Graz, Austria.
Lechner, P. & Hildenbrand, G. 1994. "Letter: Reply to Saul Green." *Townsend Letter for Doctors.* May:526–30.

p. 181    **Michael Lerner:** Lerner, M. *Choices in Healing: Integrating the Best of Conventional and Complementary Approaches to Cancer.* Cambridge, MA:MIT Press, 1994.

p. 181    **Mr. Hildenbrand:** Information presented by Mr. Hildenbrand can be found on the Center for Mind-Body Medicine's web site, located at www.cmbm.org in the 1998 CCC transcripts titled "The Dietary Treatment of Cancer (Part I)."
Hildenbrand, G., et al. 1996. "The Role of Follow-up and Retrospective Data Analysis in Alternative Cancer Management: The Gerson Experience." *J. Neuropath. Med.* 6(1):49–56.
Hildenbrand, G., et al. 1995. "Five-Year Survival Rates of Melanoma Patients Treated by Diet Therapy after the Manner of Gerson: A Retrospective Review." *Alt. Ther. Health Med.* 1(4):29–37.

p. 183   **Michio Kushi:** Kushi, M & Jack, A. *The Cancer Prevention Diet:Michio Kushi's Nutritional Blueprint for the Relief and Prevention of Disease.* New York:St. Martin's Press, 1983.

p. 184   **Dr. Lawerance Kushi:** Information presented by Dr. Kushi can be found in the 1998 CCC transcripts titled "Dietary Treatments of Cancer (Part II)" at www.cmbm.org.

p. 185   **studies have shown:** Hirayama, T. 1982. "Relationship of Soybean Paste Soup Intake to Gastric Cancer." *Nutrition and Cancer.* 3:223–33.
Teas, J., et al. 1984. "Dietary Seaweed (Laminaria) and Mammary Carcinogenesis in Rats." *Cancer Research.* 44:2758–61.
Wynder, E.L., et al. 1986. "Diet and Breast Cancer in Causation and Therapy." *Cancer.* 58:1805–11.

p. 185   **books written by cancer patients:** Sattilaro, A. *Recalled by Life.* New York: Avon Books, 1982.
Jean and Mary Alice Kohler *Healing Miracles from Macrobiotics.* Parker Publishing, 1979.

p. 187   **Dr. Block:** Information presented by Dr. Block can be found in the 1999 CCC transcripts titled "Providing Integrative Care in Office and Hospital Settings" and "Providing Integrative Care (Part I)" at www.cmbm.org.
Block, K. 1997. "The Role of the Self in Healthy Cancer Survivorship from the Front Lines of Treating Cancer." *Advances.* 13(1):6–26.

## Chapter 11: Changing the Paradigm of Cancer Care: Drs. Burzynski and Gonzalez

p. 193   **Ms. Wilkens:** Wilkens, C. "Daring to Heal My Cancer with Nutrition." *Alternative Medicine Digest.* 6:4–6.

p. 194   **Dr. Stansilaw Burzynski:** The Burzynski Research Institute's Web site is http://www.cancermed.com/.
Information on Dr. Burzynski can be found in the 1998 CCC transcripts titled, "Antineoplastons" at www.cmbm.org.
Elias, T. B. 1997. *The Burzynski Breakthrough.* Los Angeles: General Publishing Group.

p. 196   **'best case series':** Information on the best case series process can be found in the 1999 CCC transcripts titled, "The NCI Best Case Series Process" at www.cmbm.org.

p. 198   **Dr. Li-Chuan Chen:** Information presented by Dr. Chen can be found in the 1998 CCC transcripts titled, "Antineoplastons" at www.cmbm.org.

p. 198   **Dr. Arnold Eggers:** ibid.

p. 198    Dr. Robert Burdick: ibid.

p. 199    Dr. Robert Newman and Dr. Dieter Schellinger: ibid.

p. 200    Dr. Nicholas Gonzalez: Information presented by Dr. Gonzalez in the 1998 CCC transcripts titled, "Trophoblastic Hormones and Cancer: A Breakthrough in Treatment" and in the 1999 CCC transcripts titled, "Providing Integrative Care in Hospital Settings (Part I)" and "NCI/NCCAM Complementary and Alternative Medicine Clinical Trails" at www.cmbm.org.
Maver, R. W. 1991. "Nutrition and Cancer: The Gonzalez Study." *On the Risk*. 7(2).
Mitchell, T. "The War on Cancer: One Physician Is Winning, Dr. Nicholas Gonzalez." *Life Extension Practitioner*. 16–22.

p. 202    pilot study from 1994 to 1996: Gonzalez, N. J., Isaacs, L. L. 1999. "Evaluation of Pancreatic Proteolytic Enzyme Treatment of Adenocarcinoma of the Pancreas, with Nutrition and Detoxification Support." *Nutrition and Cancer*. 33(2):117–124.

p. 203    Dr. John Beard: Beard, J. 1911. *The Enzyme Treatment of Cancer*. London: Chatto and Windus.
Beard, J. 1906. "The Action of Trypsin upon the Living Cells of Jensen's Mouse Tumor." *British Medical Journal* 4:140–141.

p. 204    *Merck Manual:* Gerson, M. 1978. "The Cure of Advanced Cancer by Diet Therapy: A Summary of 30 Years of Clinical Experimentation." *Physiological Chemistry and Physics*. 10:4499–44964. Cited in U.S. Congress Office of Technology Assessment. 1990. "Unconventional Cancer Treatments." Washington DC: Government Printing Office, 46.

p. 205    recent article: Okie, S. January 18, 2000. "Maverick Treatments Find U.S. Funding." *Washington Post*. A10.

## Chapter 12: Next Steps-Dr. Fair's Tumor

p. 209    Dr. William Fair: Information presented by Dr. Fair can be found in the 1998 CCC transcripts titled, "New Therapies for Prostate Cancer," and in the 1999 CCC transcripts titled "Colon Cancer" at www.cmbm.org.

p. 210    article in the *New Yorker:* Groopman, J. October 26 and November 2, 1998. "Dr. Fair's Tumor." *The New Yorker*, 78–82, 100–106.

p. 211    Commonweal in California: Commonweal's Web site is www.commonweal.org.
Lerner, M. 1994. *Choices in Healing: Integrating the Best of Conventional and Complimentary Approaches to Cancer*. Cambridge, MA: MIT Press.

p. 213    **Stephen Jay Gould:** Gould, Stephan Jay. *Bully for Brontosauras: Reflections in Natural History.* New York: W. W. Norton and Company.

p. 216    **Spiegel:** Spiegel, D. 1994. *Living Beyond Limits: A Scientific Mind-Body Approach to Facing Life-Threatening Illness.* New York: Fawcett.

p. 216    **Fawzy:** Fawzy, F., et al. 1993. "Malignant Melanoma: Effects of an Early Structured Psychiatric Intervention, Coping, and Affective State on Recurrence and Survival 6 Years Later." *Archives of General Psychiatry.* 50:681–689.

# Bibliography

ONCE CANCER BECOMES part of our lives, many of us feel ill-prepared for and poorly informed about the decisions and choices we must make. Even a decision to do whatever a doctor—or other expert—suggests is a choice. The choice of doctor and hospital, the timing and course of treatment, as well as the selection of alternative and complementary approaches are all important decisions. Physicians and other caregivers are usually our major source of health information and treatment guidance. However, making informed choices is likely to require diligent exploration of other sources as well.

There is no single correct way to make the choices, big and small, that cancer requires. Sometimes a little guidance and information is enough; sometimes a great deal is necessary.

This bibliography is by no means complete and is intended to offer suggestions about some available and useful resources. Reading is one important way of gathering information. We hope the books discussed here will help enhance your understanding and give you the perspectives and data which will make hard choices easier.

## Integrative Approaches to Cancer

*Alternative Medicine: Expanding Medical Horizons*. (A Report to the National Institutes of Health on Alternative Medical Systems and Practices in the United States.) (NIH Publ. No. 94–006). Washington, DC: U.S. Government Printing Office, 1994.

The work of over 200 contributors and an editorial board, this book is a comprehensive compilation and evaluation of the research on a variety of alternative medical approaches. It is dense and difficult going at times, but an invaluable reference work. There is a section on pharmacological and biological treatments that discusses several alternative treatments for cancer. The sections covering research on diet and nutrition, manipulative therapies, and mind-body approaches are also useful.

Benjamin, Harold H. *The Wellness Community Guide to Fighting for Recovery from Cancer.* New York: Putnam, 1995.

This practical and reassuring book provides information on the emotional and social support that cancer patients need. Wellness communities around the country have provided guidance to more than 20,000 people with cancer.

Boik, John. *Cancer and Natural Medicine: A Textbook of Basic Science and Clinical Research*. Princeton, MN: Oregon Medical Press, 1995.
This is a fine introduction to the biology of cancer and the ways in which nutritional and herbal approaches exercise their therapeutic effects. It is comprehensive and well grounded in science.

Diamond, W. John, and W. Lee Cowden, with Burton Goldberg. *An Alternative Medicine Definitive Guide to Cancer*. Tibourn, CA: Future Medicine Publishing, Inc., 1997.
This survey of CAM treatments for cancer includes protocols of 23 "alternative" therapies plus a discussion of detection and prevention. The information and the format are interesting, with icons and clear definitions of terms, but the lack of criticism in its assessments diminishes the value of the book.

Elias, Thomas B. *The Burzynski Breakthrough*. Los Angeles: General Publishing Group, 1997.
This highly sympathetic book explores Dr. Burzynski's development and use of antineoplastons and presents a somewhat partisan view of his struggles with regulatory agencies.

Gaynor, Mitchell. *Healing Essence: A Cancer Doctor's Practical Program for Hope and Recovery*. New York: Kodansha, 1995.
This is a useful and inspiring look at the way one oncologist includes nutritional, mind-body, and spiritual approaches in his work.

Geffen, Jeremy. *The Journey Through Cancer*. New York: Crown, 2000.
A practicing oncologist's perspective on integrative care, this book is particularly strong on the importance of emotional and psychological support and on the spiritual dimensions of cancer care.

Gerson, Max. *A Cancer Therapy: Results of Fifty Cases*. Bonita, CA: Gerson Institute, 1986.
This description of Gerson's work on cancer reveals both some remarkable recoveries and questionable research.

Hersh, Stephen P. *Beyond Miracles: Living with Cancer*. Lincolnwood, IL: Contemporary Books, 1998.
This book focuses on the impact of cancer diagnosis and encourages readers to be active participants in their treatment. Discussion of treatment options includes both alternative and traditional methods.

Hess, David. *Evaluating Alternative Cancer Therapies*. New Brunswick, NJ: Rutgers University Press.
This is an overview of some of the people—and their practices—who are using, studying, and advocating for alternative therapies for cancer.

Hirshberg, Caryle, and Marc Ian Barasch. *Remarkable Recovery: What Extraordinary Healings Tell Us About Getting Well and Staying Well.* New York: Riverhead/Putnam, 1995.

This wonderful and inspiring book is based on case histories of people who recovered from apparently fatal illnesses, including, most particularly, metastatic cancer. The book emphasizes the importance of attitude, faith, and human support in the face of overwhelming odds.

Kushi, Michio. *The Cancer Prevention Diet.* New York: St. Martin's Press, 1993.

This is a discussion of the principles and practices of macrobiotics and how they can be used to prevent and treat cancer. Many of the prescriptions are excellent, and the anecdotes impressive, although, as we have noted, the scientific evidence for the efficacy of this diet in treating cancer is not available.

Lerner, Michael. *Choices in Healing: Integrating the Best of Conventional and Complementary Approaches to Cancer.* Cambridge, MA: MIT Press, 1994.

An extremely thoughtful and valuable overview of alternative cancer therapies, this is "must reading" for anyone with cancer.

LeShan, Lawrence. *Cancer as a Turning Point.* Rev. ed. New York: Penguin Group, 1994.

Psychological change provides hope for mobilizing a compromised immune system. For 35 years, LeShan has worked with cancer patients. The structure of this "handbook" blends anecdotes with professional advice and includes a workbook to help enhance physical and psychological health by improving and enriching life choices.

Moss, Ralph W. *Cancer Therapy.* Brooklyn, NY: Equinox Press, Inc., 1992.

The subtitle says it: "Consumer's Guide to Non-Toxic Treatment and Prevention." Moss discusses over 100 alternative treatments for cancer, with documentation from the scientific literature. His aim is to provide useful information on cancer treatment alternatives and to encourage freedom of choice for cancer patients.

Pelton, Ross, and Lee Overholser. *Alternatives in Cancer Therapy.* New York: Fireside, 1994.

This is a well-researched, if not sufficiently critical, guide to some of the more widely used alternative treatments.

Porter, Garrett, and Patricia Norris. *Why Me?* Walpole, NH: Stillpoint, 1985.

This is an inspiring account of the power of the healing partnership and the skillful use of imagery to heal a young boy with brain cancer.

Siegel, Bernie. *Love, Medicine, and Miracles: Lessons Learned About Self-Healing from a Surgeon's Experience with Exceptional Patients.* New York: HarperCollins, 1986.

This best-seller by a Yale surgeon has helped many people to realize that they can be "exceptions" to the grim statistics that often confront patients with cancer and other life-threatening illnesses,

Walters, Richard. *Options: The Alternative Cancer Therapy Book*. Garden City Park, NY: Avery, 1993.

This is a useful if somewhat outdated overview of a number of alternative approaches.

## Basic Information and References on Cancer

Bazell, Robert. *Her–2*. New York: Random House, 1998.

Herceptin is the first treatment targeted at a gene defect giving rise to breast cancer. This is the story of the drug, so far, and of the politics, money, and science that influence medical research. It is also about the heroic women who volunteered for clinical trials.

Berkow, Robert, ed. *The Merck Manual of Medical Information*. Whitehouse Station, NJ: Merck Research Laboratories, 1997.

This is an instant resource for summaries on health issues.

Bernstein, Peter L. *Against the Gods: The Remarkable Story of Risk*. New York: John Wiley and Sons, Inc., 1996.

Bernstein, president of an economic consulting firm, delves into the idea of risk and the need to control chance in our lives.

Bognar, David. *CANCER: Increasing Your Odds for Survival*. Alameda, CA: Hunter House Publishers, 1998.

This is a good resource guide for people with cancer. It covers both conventional and alternative therapies and uses both information from acknowledged experts and the experience of patients.

Dollinger, Malin, Ernest Rosenbaum, and Greg Cable. *Everyone's Guide to Cancer Therapy*. Rev. 3d ed. Kansas City, MO: Andrew McMeel Publishing, 1997.

The third edition is a readable and authoritative reference work on cancer from the best conventional sources, including the National Cancer Institute.

Gould, Stephen Jay. *Bully for Brontosaurus: Reflections in Natural History*. New York: W. W. Norton and Company, 1991.

This is a collection of Gould's enlightening scientific essays.

Hall, Stephen S. *A Commotion in the Blood*. New York: Henry Holt and Company. 1997.

This is a fascinating narrative about the development of immunotherapy, from Coley's toxins through new genetic discoveries. Hall follows the story of how much we know, and don't know, about the immune system. This is science writing at its best, dazzling and informative.

Keene, Nancy. *Childhood Leukemia*. Sebastopal, CA: O'Reilly and Associates, 1997.

> The illness and treatment of children has special problems for patient, family, and other caregivers. This matter-of-fact book combines personal experience and interviews with solid medical information. Throughout, the emphasis is on what "works," a practical guide through the devastating reality of childhood leukemia.

Love, Susan M. *Dr. Susan Love's Breast Book*. 2d ed. Reading, MA: Perseus Books, 1995.

> This is a fine reference book on breast care, including screening, diagnosis, treatment, and research. Dr. Love is a straightforward and concise writer; her knowledge, thoughtfulness, and caring are obvious on every page.

Morra, Marion, and Eve Potts. *Choices*. Rev. ed. New York: Avon Books, 1994.

> This is a good, basic reference guide to cancer diagnosis and treatment. It includes information on procedures, diagnostic technologies, and new research on therapies.

Morra, Marion, and Eve Potts. *The Prostate Cancer Answer Book: An Unbiased Guide to Treatment Choices*. New York: Avon Books, 1996.

> This book provides a detailed look at prostate cancer, from characteristics of the illness itself to treatment options.

Riegelman, Richard K., and Robert P. Hirsch. *Studying a Study and Testing a Test*. 3d ed. New York: Little, Brown and Company, 1996.

> If one has a science background, or wants to understand scientific literature, this is *the* book. It is written for medical students and professionals, carefully explaining how to read journal articles more critically and efficiently. It also includes a complete glossary.

Weinberg, Robert A. *One Renegade Cell: How Cancer Begins*. New York: Basic Books, 1998.

> This book tracks cancer from its biological roots to its possible cure. The author, a molecular biologist, is the director of the Oncology Research Laboratory at the Whitehead Institute.

## Integrative Medicine: General References

Benson, Herbert, and E. Stuart. *The Wellness Book: The Comprehensive Guide to Maintaining Health and Treating Stress-Related Illness*. Secaucus, NJ: Carol Publishing Group, 1992.

> This is an easy-to-read self-help guide. Each chapter focuses on a specific aspect of the mind-body approach, including exercise, nutrition, and stress management. It provides basic information and self-assessments and is full of illustrations and practical exercises.

Benson, Herbert, and Miriam Z. Klipper. *The Relaxation Response*. New York: William Morrow and Company. 1975.

This book documents the remarkable results of simple, meditative techniques in early mind-body research and treatment studies. It includes a straightforward introduction to relaxation practice.

Cassileth, Barrie. *The Alternative Medicine Handbook*. New York: W. W. Norton and Company, 1998.

An expert investigator of complementary and alternative medicine (CAM) presents her evaluation of over 50 alternative and complementary therapies. This is a careful and clearly written introduction to the scientific basis of CAM research. Not a definitive or comprehensive resource, but it is easy to read and well organized.

Chopra, Deepak. *Perfect Health*. New York: Harmony Books, 1991.

This introduction to Ayurvedic health practices (including a program of daily routines based on individual body type) has been widely read by people seeking a new understanding of health and the mind-body connection.

Dreher, Henry. *The Immune Power Personality: 7 Traits You Can Develop to Stay Healthy*. New York: Dutton, 1995.

This is a fine, comprehensive, well-written discussion of the ways in which attitude and emotion affect immune system functioning. Dreher presents the work of such researchers as George Solomon, who studied the effects of emotion on arthritis, and James Pennebaker, who explored the utility of self-expression through journal keeping.

Gordon, James S. *Holistic Medicine*. New York: Chelsea House, 1988.

This is a brief overview of the field and some of the techniques that are generally included in it.

Gordon, James S., Dennis T. Jaffe, and David E. Bresler (eds.) *Mind, Body, and Health: Toward an Integral Medicine*. New York: Human Sciences Press, 1984.

A compendium of articles on therapeutic approaches, the emphasis of this book is on pioneering programs that have been developed to address specific problems—chronic and acute pain, childbirth, aging, cancer and others—rather than on specific modalities.

Gordon, James S. *Manifesto for a New Medicine: Your Guide to Healing Partnerships and the Wise Use of Alternative Therapies*. New York: Addison-Wesley Publishing Company. 1996.

This clear, readable, eminently useful guide to a "New Medicine" which combines modern science and ancient wisdom, helps readers to see the power they have to help themselves. One chapter in particular is devoted to a patient with cancer who creates a remarkably rich program of physical, emotional, and spiritual healing.

Moyers, Bill. *Healing and the Mind*. New York: Doubleday, 1993.

This is a compilation of interviews on various aspects of the new medicine with participants in the television series of the same name. Moyers addresses common questions about techniques such as acupuncture and meditation. There is a nice section on Commonweal's work with cancer patients.

Ornish, Dean. *Dr. Dean Ornish's Program for Reversing Heart Disease Without Drugs or Surgery.* New York: Ballantine, 1992.

Ornish's program for reversing heart disease offers a good perspective on the effective use of a comprehensive mind-body approach, including nutrition and exercise, relaxation techniques, yoga, and group support. This is a wonderful example of the way in which clinical work with the mind-body approach can not only provide enormous benefits to patients but also yield positive research results.

Pelletier, Kenneth. *Mind As Healer, Mind As Slayer: A Holistic Approach to Preventing Stress Disorders.* New York: Delta, 1977.

This pioneering book offers a clear, straightforward presentation of research on the effects of stress on the human body. It is also a good summary of nonpharmacological techniques that have been used to alleviate the effects of stress, including meditation, autogenic training, and biofeedback.

Weil, Andrew. *Natural Health, Natural Medicine.* Boston: Houghton Mifflin Company, 1990.

This is a guide to health maintenance, including suggestions for the treatment of some common illnesses, utilizing self-care methods that are safe, natural, and inexpensive.

_____. *Spontaneous Healing: How to Discover and Enhance Your Body's Natural Ability to Heal Itself.* New York: Alfred A. Knopf, 1995.

This clear, well-written discussion emphasizes the power each of us has to mobilize our mind and body to heal ourselves. The book provides good, solid information and suggestions for constructive lifestyle changes.

## The Mind-Body-Spirit Connection

Achterberg, Jeanne. *Imagery in Healing: Shamanism and Modern Medicine.* Boston: New Science Library Publisher, 1985.

A research psychologist presents a thoughtful overview of how mind and culture influence the human body.

Benson, Herbert. *Timeless Healing: The Power and Biology of Belief.* New York: Fireside, 1996.

This is an exploration of the connection between religious faith and physical well-being.

Borysenko, Joan. *Fire in the Soul: A New Psychology of Spiritual Optimism.* New York: Warner Books, 1994.

Borysenko offers a very personal guide to understanding life crises as part of a process of spiritual growth.

_____. *Minding the Body, Mending the Mind*. Reading, MA: Addison-Wesley, 1987.

This is a very good, readable, and practical introduction to the mind-body approach by a cell biologist and psychologist who has done laboratory research and clinical work. Joan Borysenko has a wonderful heart as well as an organized mind, and both are apparent here.

Dossey, Larry. *Healing Words: The Power of Prayer and the Practice of Medicine*. New York: HarperCollins, 1993.

This clear, well-written overview of the power of prayer to affect people physically and emotionally is based on hundreds of published studies.

Epstein, Gerald. *Healing Visualizations: Creating Health with Imagery*. New York: Bantam, 1989.

This is a guide by a New York psychiatrist to the use of imagery in healing. Epstein is primarily a clinician rather than researcher, and this book provides many useful exercises to mobilize the mind to understand and assist the body and itself.

Goleman, Daniel. *The Meditative Mind*. Los Angeles: J. P. Tarcher, 1988.

A *New York Times* reporter offers a good overview of the world's meditative traditions, discussing some of the scientific literature on meditation.

Goleman, Daniel, and Joel Gurin, eds. *Mind/Body Medicine: How to Use Your Mind for Better Health*. Yonkers, NY: Consumer Reports Books, 1993.

In this book some of America's leading physicians, psychologists, and medical researchers write about the connection between stress and illness and a variety of mind-body approaches such as hypnosis, biofeedback, meditation, and psychotherapy.

Holland, Jimmie C., and Julia H. Rowland. *Handbook of Psychooncology: Psychological Care of the Patient with Cancer*. New York: Oxford University Press, 1989.

This technical medical text discusses how oncologists should approach cancer patients' emotional as well as physical states.

Institute of Noetic Sciences, with William Poole. *The Heart of Healing*. Atlanta, GA: Turner Publishing, 1993.

This is a nicely illustrated companion to the Institute of Noetic Sciences' series that appeared on Turner Broadcasting Systems. The emphasis of the book is on the power of the mind to affect our health, the therapeutic effect of spiritual practice, and intriguing but so-far inexplicable instances of remarkable recoveries.

Kabat-Zinn, Jon. *Full Catastrophe Living: Using the Wisdom of Your Body and Mind to Face Stress, Pain, and Illness*. New York: Dell, 1990.

This book, by the director of a comprehensive program for the treatment of chronic illness at the University of Massachusetts Medical Center, gives a sense of the attitude that pervades the program, one of "mindfulness." It shows how yoga, meditation, and group support may be used in the treatment of chronic pain, anxiety disorders, and other conditions.

Kabat-Zinn, Jon. *Wherever You Go, There You Are.* New York: Hyperion, 1994.

This is a wise guide to bringing the practice of mindfulness into everyday life by the director of the Stress Management Clinic at the University of Massachusetts Medical Center.

Kornfield, Jack. *A Path with Heart: A Guide Through the Perils and Promises of Spiritual Life.* New York: Bantam, 1993.

This is a gentle, thoughtful approach to meditative life by an American psychologist who spent years studying Buddhist practice in Southeast Asia.

Martin, Paul. *The Healing Mind.* New York: St. Martin's Press, 1997.

The past few years have brought enormous advances in our understanding of the mind-body connection. This is a fine account of the scientific research supporting what we intuitively know: that mental and emotional states affect our bodily health, that the mind and body are entirely linked.

Mitchell, Stephen. *The Enlightened Heart: An Anthology of Poetry.* New York: Harper, 1992.

This is an anthology of sacred poetry, well chosen and well translated, from the Bible, Rumi, Lao Tzu, etc. Sample: "A good traveler has no fixed plans and is not intent upon arriving. A good artist lets his intuition lead him wherever it wants. A good scientist has freed himself of concepts and keeps his mind open to what is"—Lao Tzu.

Moore, Thomas. *Care of the Soul: A Guide for Cultivating Depth and Sacredness in Everyday Life.* New York: HarperCollins, 1992.

Moore has written a lovely and popular book on the spiritual dimension of health and healing.

Nhat Hanh, Thich. *The Miracle of Mindfulness: A Manual on Meditation.* Boston: Beacon Press, 1987. (Originally published in 1975.)

_____. *Peace Is Every Step: The Path of Mindfulness in Everyday Life.* New York: Bantam, 1991.

These are wonderful, practical books by a Vietnamese Buddhist monk. The techniques of mindfulness meditation are taught by many practitioners and are integrated practice in programs in major cancer centers.

Pert, Candace. *Molecules of Emotion.* New York: Scribner, 1997.

This is the fascinating story of the research scientist who discovered some of the biochemical underpinnings of the mind-body connection.

Spiegel, David. *Living Beyond Limits: A Scientific Mind-Body Approach to Facing Life-Threatening Illness.* New York: Fawcett, 1994.

The emphasis in this popular account of Spiegel's work with women with metastatic breast cancer is on the power of psychological support and self-expression to affect well-being and outcome.

## Diet, Nutrition, and Herbs

Arnot, Bob. *The Breast Cancer Prevention Diet*. New York: Little, Brown & Company, 1998.
This book presents some of the recent studies on the possible relationship between diet and breast cancer and suggests a program of dietary changes to prevent recurrences.

Atkins, Robert C. *Dr. Atkins' New Diet Revolution*. New York: Avon Books, Inc., 1992.
Being overweight is a risk factor in many chronic diseases, including cancer. Dr. Atkins promotes a low-carbohydrate, high-protein diet that is easy to follow. Other researchers studying connections between diet and cancer are exploring similar metabolic processes.

Balch, James F., and Phyllis A. Balch. *Prescription for Nutritional Healing*. Garden City Park, NY: Avery, 1990.
This is a self-help guide to nutritional supplements and their therapeutic use. Unfortunately, it's not well-referenced.

Bland, Jeffrey, with Sarah Bemum. *Genetic Nutritioneering*. Los Angeles, Keats: 1999.
A fascinating discussion of the way foods and supplements can affect the expression of genes. This is extremely useful information on foods that may contribute to cancer prevention.

Duke, James, and S. Foster. *Peterson's Field Guide to Medicinal Plants*. Boston: Houghton-Mifflin, 1990.
One of the world's leading authorities on medicinal herbs offers this lavishly illustrated guide to their use.

Golan, Ralph. *Optimal Wellness*. New York: Bantam, 1995.
A family physician gives an excellent introduction to the use of natural therapies for health promotion and the treatment of illness. This book has very strong and practical sections on food allergies, hypoglycemia, nutritional deficiencies, and "dietary hazards and excesses."

Haas, Elson M. *Staying Healthy with Nutrition: The Complete Guide to Diet and Nutritional Medicine*. Berkeley, CA: Celestial Arts, 1992.
This is a fine overview of nutrition and of the use of nutritional therapies for specific illnesses.

Haas, Robert. *Permanent Remissions*. New York: Pocket Books, 1997.
This book offers nutritional information and recipes for the therapeutic use of phytonutrients.

Moss, Ralph W. *Antioxidants Against Cancer*. New York: Equinox Press, 2000. A painstakingly referenced and practical survey of the scientific evidence for antioxidant's in comprehensive cancer care.

_____. *Herbs Against Cancer*. New York: Equinox, 1998.
Science writer and patient advocate Moss presents a review of the history of—and controversy surrounding—the use of herbs in the treatment of cancer.

Nixon, Daniel W. *The Cancer Recovery Eating Plan.* New York: Random House, 1994.
This excellent book covers much of what we know about the link between cancer and nutrition. Dr. Nixon emphasizes individualized eating plans and ways to increase comfort during treatment.

Simone, Charles. *Cancer and Nutrition.* Garden City Park, NY: Avery, 1994.
This is an oncologist's overview of the role of nutrition in the prevention and treatment of cancer, together with useful guidelines for eating and supplementation.

Yance, Donald. *Herbal Medicine: Healing and Cancer.* Chicago, IL: Keats, 1999.
A practicing herbalist gives a broad and useful review of herbal treatments and how they may be able to inhibit the growth and spread of cancer.

## Exploring Chinese Medicine

Beinfield, Harriet, and Efrem Korngold. *Between Heaven and Earth: A Guide to Chinese Medicine.* New York: Ballantine, 1991.
This is probably the best and most complete introduction to the philosophy of Chinese medicine and acupuncture. It also gives a nice sense of how another culture views mind and body as inseparable and approaches illness in a more holistic way.

Bensky, Dan, and Andrew Gamble. *Chinese Herbal Medicine: Materia Medica.* Rev. ed. Seattle: Eastland Press, 1993.
This comprehensive text discusses the traditional uses of Chinese herbs and the modern scientific evidence that justifies these uses.

Cohen, Kenneth S. *The Way of Qigong: The Art and Science of Chinese Energy Healing.* New York: Ballantine, 1997.
The author, who studied extensively in China, has written an excellent introduction to the theory, practice, and research on both internal and external *qi gong*.

Eisenberg, David S., with Thomas Lee Wright. *Encounters with Qi: Exploring Chinese Medicine.* New York: Penguin Books, 1987.
This is an account of Chinese medicine and particularly of the communication of qi from healers to patients. The author is an American physician who studied and traveled widely in China.

Frantzis, B. K. *Opening the Energy Gates of Your Body.* Berkeley, CA: North Atlantic Books, 1993.
*Qigong* exercises are explained as a means of opening up the body's energy channels.

Gevitz, Norman, ed. *Other Healers: Unorthodox Medicine in America.* Baltimore: Johns Hopkins University Press, 1988.

This is an introduction to the history of other medical treatments in the United States.

Hammer, Leon. *Dragon Rises, Red Bird Flies: Psychology & Chinese Medicine.* Barrytown, NY: Station Hill Press, 1990.

A psychiatrist and teacher of TCM offers a wise and comprehensive treatment of the five-element approach to Chinese medicine. The emphasis is on psychological issues and the utility of the five elements as a way of understanding and explaining behavior. Also discussed are the difficulty of integrating Traditional Chinese Medicine and scientific medical research and the ways each may change each other.

Kaptchuk, Ted. *The Web That Has No Weaver: Understanding Chinese Medicine.* Chicago: Contemporary Books, 1985.

This is an extremely useful introduction to the spirit and substance of traditional Chinese medicine by an American who studied in Macao and teaches at Harvard Medical School.

Reid, Daniel. *The Complete Book of Chinese Health and Healing.* Boston: Shambhala, 1995.

A good overview of the various aspects of Chinese medicine, this book is particularly strong in its discussion of *qi gong.*

Sobel, David S. *Ways of Health: Holistic Approaches to Ancient and Contemporary Medicine.* New York: Harcourt Brace Jovanovich, 1979.

This extremely useful survey of other medical traditions includes some of the most telling critiques of Western medicine as well as snapshots from Hippocratic, Chinese, and American Indian sources.

## Personal Experience

Cousins, Norman. *Anatomy of an Illness.* New York: W. W. Norton and Company, 1979.

Although this book was written over 20 years ago, it carries a message of power and hope. Cousins was one of the first to articulate a model of healing partnership between physician and patient and to recognize the potency of consciously utilizing the mind to affect the body.

French, Marilyn. *A Season in Hell.* New York: Alfred A. Knopf, 1998.

This memoir, by a writer known for her provocative intelligence and sometimes shocking honesty, is about French's struggle with esophageal cancer. French's ability to focus on life and living enables her to defy a dismal prognosis.

Landro, Laura. *Survivor.* New York: Simon and Schuster, 1998.

*Survivor* is a manifesto for the need to inform oneself to survive cancer. For Landro, knowledge was inseparable from successful treatment.

Lipsyte, Robert. *In the Country of Illness*. New York: Alfred A. Knopf, 1998.
Lipsyte gives helpful advice on coping with cancer, concentrating your energies on what matters, and ways to deal with unhelpful bureaucrats. This account of his own and his ex-wife's cancer also offers a picture of grace and humor in the face of devastating illness.

Price, Reynolds. *A Whole New Life: An Illness and a Healing*. New York: Penguin, 1995.
Catastrophic illness rarely improves one's character; for the novelist Reynolds Price, it becomes a gift of life. More than a memoir of illness, this is the story of a deeply spiritual struggle.

Rollin, Betty. *First, You Cry*. New York: The New American Library, 1976.
In 1974, no one talked about breast cancer. Rollin, along with Betty Ford and Happy Rockefeller, broke the silence and in the process began to change breast cancer care and research. Truly a pioneering book, it still stands as an intimate and honest story of the effect of breast cancer on one woman's life.

Sarton, May. *A Reckoning*. New York: W. W. Norton & Company, 1978.
This enlightening novel follows a woman diagnosed with terminal cancer as she chooses how to "live her dying."

Winawer, Sidney. *Healing Lessons*. New York: Little, Brown & Company, 1998.
The transformative power of a cancer diagnosis is becoming part of our understanding of catastrophic illness. Here, a distinguished oncologist is educated and humbled by the illness and death of his wife.

# Index